ECG Simplified
Facts You Will Never Forget

ECG Simplified
Facts You Will Never Forget

David C Barold, MD
S Serge Barold, MD

Conductivity
Press

First Edition

Copyright © 2022 by Conductivity Press, Inc

Conductivity Press, Inc
900 La Fiesta Way
San Marcos, CA 92078

Comments, inquiries, and requests for bulk sales can be directed to the publisher at: info@conductivitypress.com

All rights reserved. No part of this publication may be reproduced, distributed, or transmitted in any form or by any means, including photocopying, recording, or other electronic or mechanical methods, without the prior written permission of the publisher, except in the case of brief quotations embodied in critical articles and reviews. For permission requests, please contact Conductivity Press at permissions@conductivitypress.com.

This book is not intended as a substitute for the medical recommendation of physicians or other health-care providers. The publisher does not provide medical advice or guidance and this work is merely a reference tool. Health-care professionals, and not the publisher, are solely responsible for the use of this work including all medical judgements and for any resulting diagnosis and treatments.

ISBN Number: 978-1-7362045-5-9

Library of Congress Control Number: 2021909503

Printed in USA

Table of Contents

PART 1 - BASICS   1

Chapter 1 - Basic Anatomy and Physiology   2
The Heart Is a Pump   3
The Cardiac Cycle   5
The Myocardium   6
Myocardial Cell Up Close   7
Conduction System of the Heart   10
Normal Activation of the Heart   12

Chapter 2 - Origin of the Electrocardiogram   15
What is an Electrocardiogram   16
How Electrical Signals Are Detected   17
Brief History of the Electrocardiogram   18
Dipole Theory   20
Vectors   21
Waveform Deflections   22

Chapter 3 - ECG Leads   27
12 Different Viewpoints   28
Frontal Plane Lead Systems   29
    Standard Limb Leads
    Augmented Leads
    Frontal Plane Hexaxial Diagram
Transverse Plane Lead System   38
Views of the Heart and Corresponding Leads   40
12-Lead ECG Format   41
12-Lead ECG Recording Procedure   42

Chapter 4 - ECG Waveforms, Axis and Intervals   43
ECG Paper   44
Isoelectric Line   46
ECG Waveforms   47
P wave   48
QRS Complex   50
    Origin of the QRS Complex
    QRS Width
    QRS Axis (Frontal plane axis)
T Wave   61
ST Segment   63
ECG Intervals   64
Sinus Rhythm   72
Normal ECG Measurements   74

PART 2 - MORPHOLOGICAL ABNORMALITIES 75

Chapter 5 - Atrial Abnormalities 76
Left Atrial Abnormality 77
Right Atrial Abnormality 78

Chapter 6 - Ventricular Hypertrophy 79
Left Ventricular Hypertrophy 80
Right Ventricular Hypertrophy 84

Chapter 7 - Intraventricular Conduction Disturbances 85
Right Bundle Branch Block 86
Left Bundle Branch Block 91
Left Anterior Fascicular Block 97
Left Posterior Fascicular Block 101
Bifascicular Block 105

Chapter 8 - Myocardial Ischemia and Infarction 109
Myocardial Ischemia 110
ST Elevation Myocardial Infarction 112
Non-ST Elevation Myocardial Infarction and Unstable Angina 120
Pathological Q Waves 125
Myocardial Infarction and Bundle Branch Block 128

Chapter 9 - Other Causes of ST Elevation 129
Early Repolarization 130
Pericarditis 132
Left Ventricular Aneurysm 134
Brugada Syndrome 135
Concave vs Convex Patterns of ST Elevation 136

PART 3 - RHYTHM DISTURBANCES 137

Chapter 10 - Atrial and Junctional Rhythms 139
Sinus Bradycardia 140
Sinus Arrhythmia 141
Sinoatrial Exit Block 142
Sinus Arrest 143
Atrial Premature Complexes 144
Wandering Atrial Pacemaker 147
Junctional Arrhythmias 148
Junctional Premature Complex
Junctional Rhythms

Chapter 11 - Supraventricular Tachyarrhythmias   153
Sinus Tachycardia   154
Focal Atrial Tachycardia   155
Multifocal Atrial Tachycardia   157
Atrial Fibrillation   158
Atrial Flutter   162
AV Nodal Reentrant Tachycardia   165
AV Reentrant Tachycardia   169
Sick Sinus Syndrome   171
Evaluation of a Narrow QRS Complex Tachycardia   172

Chapter 12 - Wolf Parkinson White Syndrome   174

Chapter 13 - Ventricular Arrhythmias   180
Ventricular Premature Complexes   181
Ventricular Escape Rhythm   186
Accelerated Idioventricular Rhythm   187

Chapter 14 - Ventricular Tachyarrhythmias   189
Ventricular Tachycardia   190
Wide QRS Complex Tachycardia   195
Ventricular Flutter   196
Ventricular Fibrillation   197

Chapter 15 - Atrioventricular Conduction Blocks   199
First Degree AV Block   200
Second Degree AV Block   201
     Type I
     Type II
     2:1
     Advanced
     Pitfalls In The Diagnosis of Type II AV Block
Third Degree AV Block   210
AV Dissociation   212

PART 4 - MISCELLANEOUS ECG ABNORMALITIES   215

Chapter 16 - Miscellaneous ECG Abnormalities   215
Hyperkalemia   216
Hypokalemia   217
Pulmonary Embolism   218
Low Voltage   219
Electrical Alternans   220
Pacemaker   221
ECG Electrode Misplacement   227
Artifact and Pseudoarrhythmias   228

PART 5 - HOW TO READ AN ECG 229

PART 6 - APPENDICES 241

    Appendix A: Further Reading 241

INDEX 243

Preface

Learning ECG interpretation is not easy. Therefore, we set out to write a book on basic electrocardiography emphasizing visuals to facilitate learning, understanding and retention of key facts. Consequently, *ECG Simplified* contains an extensive collection of graphic illustrations supported by concise text. This format provides *ECG Simplified* with facts easy to remember. We have restricted our mission to straight electrocardiography as a basis for further learning of pathophysiology and therapy found in more advanced texts. Although the book was intended to educate beginners without previous knowledge of electrocardiography, its potential benefit should not be overlooked by more knowledgeable individuals who might find it a useful resource to rapidly refresh their skills in ECG interpretation. The book is accompanied by more than 100 practice questions available online (www.ECGSimplified.com).

David & Serge

Companion Website

This book is accompanied by practice tests for each part of the book to evaluate your acquired knowledge. These self-assessment tests are available on the following companion website:

www.ECGSimplified.com

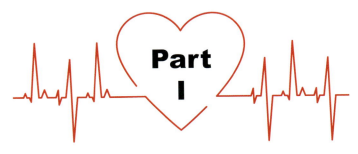

Part I

Basics

Basic Anatomy & Physiology of the Heart

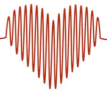

The Heart Is A Pump

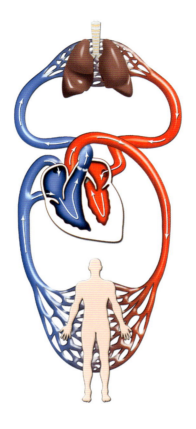

The heart lies at the center of the circulatory system and is responsible for pumping blood throughout the body. The heart actually consists of two pumps. The **right-sided pump** receives deoxygenated blood from the body and delivers it to the lungs to be oxygenated. The **left-sided pump** receives the oxygenated blood from the lungs and delivers it to the body. The right- and left-sided pumps are separated by a wall called the **septum**. Each of these pumps is comprised of two chambers, the **atrium** and the **ventricle**.

When the deoxygenated blood arrives to the heart, it first enters the **right atrium** from two large veins, the **superior** and **inferior vena cava**. The right atrium contracts, propelling the blood into the **right ventricle** via the **tricuspid valve**. After a period of relaxation for ventricular filling of blood, the right ventricle contracts, propelling blood through the **pulmonary valve** into the pulmonary circulation where oxygenation in the lungs takes place.

The **left atrium** receives the oxygenated blood from the lungs and contracts, propelling the blood into the **left ventricle** via the **mitral valve**. After a period of relaxation for ventricular filling of blood, the left ventricle contracts, propelling blood into the **aorta** via the **aortic valve**.

The right- and left-sided pumps contract simultaneously.

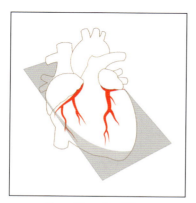

Four Chamber View

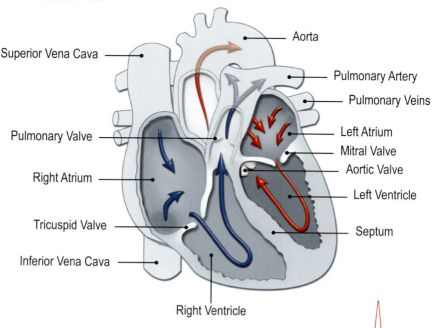

The Cardiac Cycle

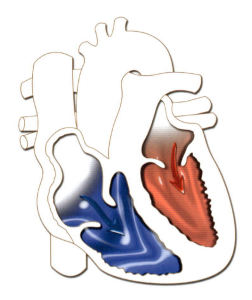 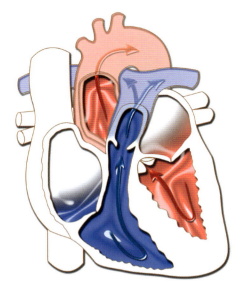

Ventricular Diastole (Relaxation)   Ventricular Systole (Contraction)

Within each cardiac cycle, there are two phases. During **ventricular diastole**, the ventricles are relaxed, allowing infilling of blood into the ventricular chambers from the contracted atria. During **ventricular systole**, the ventricles contract, propelling blood into the lungs and body via the arterial system.

The Myocardium

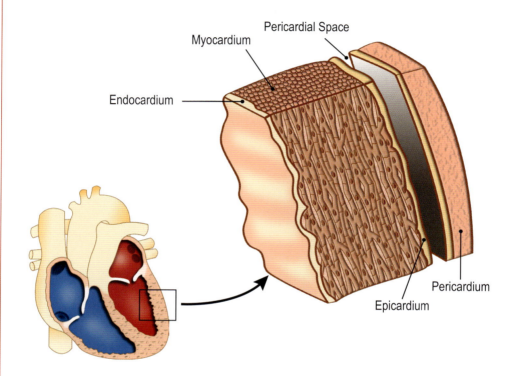

The **myocardium**, the middle layer of the heart, forms the bulk of the heart. It is sandwiched between the **endocardium** (inner layer of the wall of the heart) and the **epicardium** (outer protective layer of the heart). The **epicardium** is also the innermost layer of the **pericardium** (fibroelastic sac enclosing the heart).

Within the myocardium are millions of interconnected and interlacing bundles of electrically excitable muscle fibers (**myocardial contractile cells**) that enable the heart to contract.

Myocardial Cell Up Close

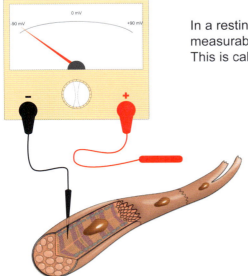

In a resting state, a myocardial contractile cell has a measurable voltage across its membrane of -90 mV. This is called the **resting membrane potential**.

Voltage is the electrical potential difference between 2 different points and is measured using a voltmeter.

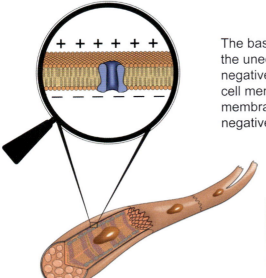

The basis of the resting membrane potential is the unequal distribution of positive and negative ions (Na, K, Cl and Ca) across the cell membrane resulting in the outside of the membrane being positive and inside being negative.

When there is this separation of charge, the membrane is described as being "polarized".

7

When the myocardial cell encounters an electrical impulse, there is a sudden redistribution of ions resulting in **depolarization** or loss of the difference in the charge between the inside and outside of the cell. This is followed briefly by a reversal of the polarity (outside negative and inside positive) resulting in the membrane potential becoming slightly positive.

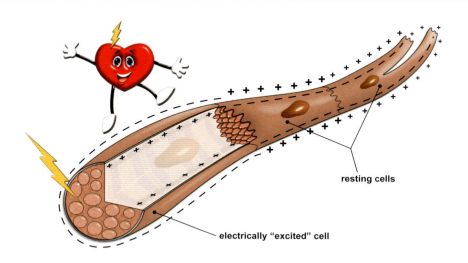

What follows is **repolarization**, the gradual return back to the resting membrane potential of -90 mV. The cardiac action potential depicts the changes of the membrane potential during the depolarization and the subsequent repolarization of the cell.

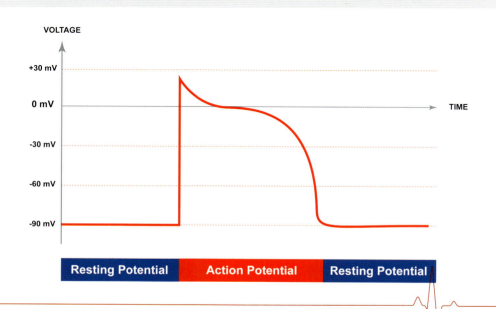

Current generated from the cell membrane during these voltage fluctuations triggers this excitable activity in the membranes of neighboring cardiac cells and a domino effect occurs resulting in a depolarization "wave" that spreads rapidly throughout the muscle tissue.

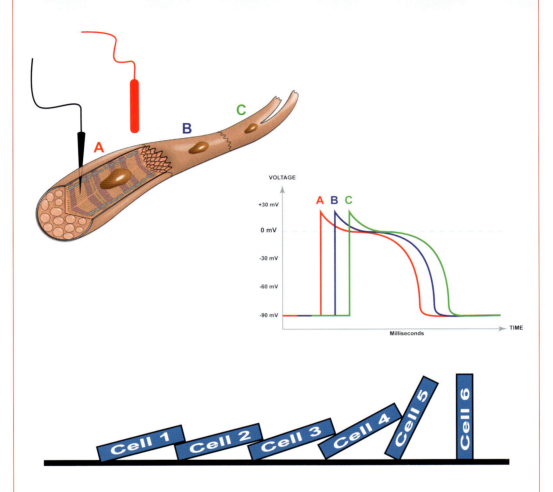

Cardiac muscle behaves as a functional syncytium. Once all of cardiac cells in the atria or ventricle are depolarized, they function as a coordinated unit and contract almost in unison.

Conduction System of the Heart

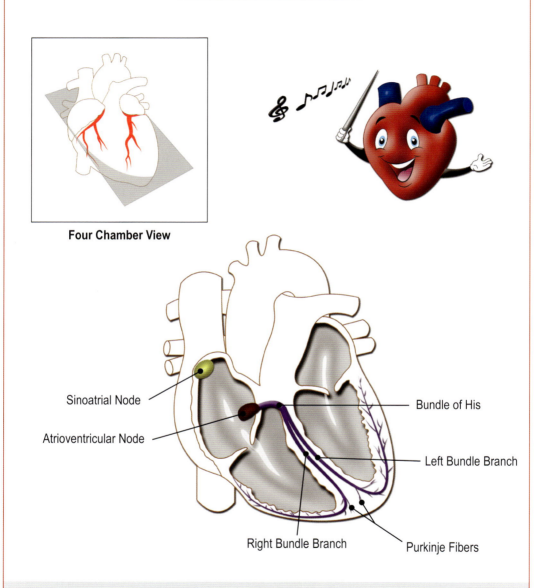

Four Chamber View

- Sinoatrial Node
- Atrioventricular Node
- Bundle of His
- Left Bundle Branch
- Right Bundle Branch
- Purkinje Fibers

The above diagram depicts the network of highly specialized cells within the myocardium (**myocardial conducting cells**) whose function is to generate and coordinate the electrical activity of the heart to allow for pump efficiency. It ensures that the atria contract before the ventricles and the right and left sides of the heart operate in synchrony.

Conduction System in the Left Ventricle

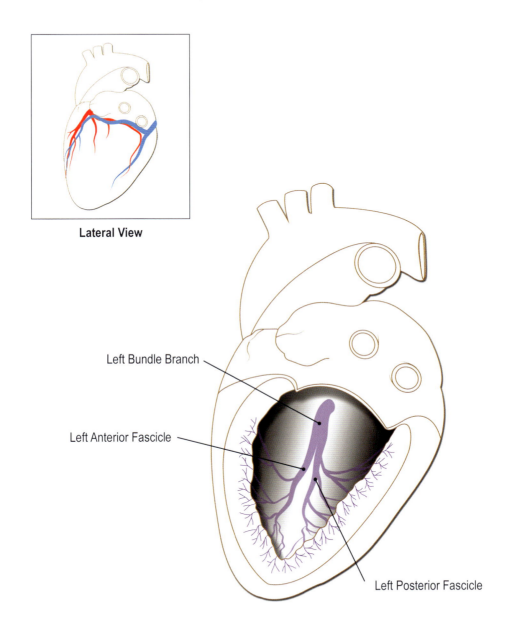

The left bundle branch bifurcates into the left anterior and left posterior fascicles. The right bundle branch does not bifurcate.

Normal Activation Sequence of the Heart

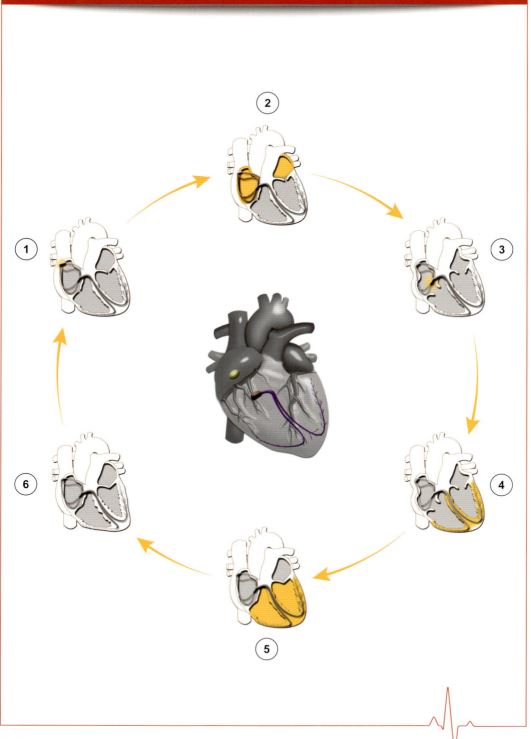

Normal activation sequence of the heart:

 The **sinoatrial (SA) node** generates the electrical impulse.

 The impulse spreads throughout the right and left atria (atrial depolarization). Atrial contraction follows atrial depolarization.

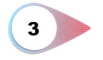 The impulse then reaches the **atrioventricular (AV) node**, the only connection between the atria and ventricles in the normal heart. Conduction of the impulse slows considerably in the AV node introducing a delay between atrial and ventricular activation. This ensures that the atria fully contract and propel blood into the ventricle before the ventricles contract.

> In disease states when conduction from the atria to the ventricles is completely interrupted, complete AV block intervenes where upon the atria and the ventricles beat independently of each other. In partial AV block, the number of conducted atrial impulses are expressed as a ratio. For example, 2:1 block means that every other atrial impulse is conducted to the ventricle.

 The impulse is rapidly conducted down the **bundle of His** (often referred to as the His bundle) then down the **right** and **left bundle branches** and eventually the **Purkinje fibers** which interface with the left and right ventricular myocardial contractile cells.

 The impulse spreads throughout the right and left ventricles (ventricular depolarization).

 Ventricular contraction follows ventricular depolarization.

> It takes less than 0.20 seconds for an electrical impulse to travel from the SA node to the ventricular myocardial cells in a normal heart.

13

Conduction of an impulse in the normal direction from the SA node to the ventricles is referred to as anterograde (forward) conduction. Conduction occurring in the opposite direction from the ventricles or AV node to the atria is referred to as retrograde (reverse) conduction and is often abnormal.

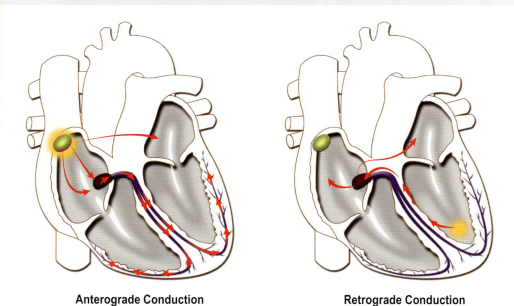

Anterograde Conduction **Retrograde Conduction**

In case the SA node fails to generate an impulse, the heart has a back up system. Listed here are tissues that can assume pacemaker activity, though at a slower rate.

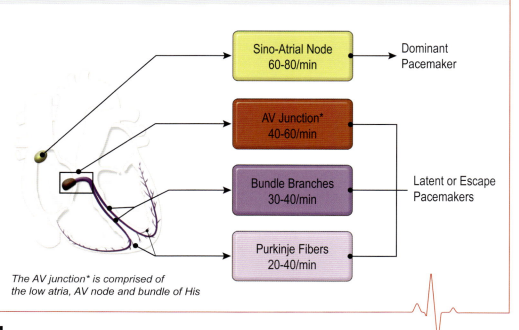

The AV junction* is comprised of the low atria, AV node and bundle of His

Origin of the Electrocardiogram

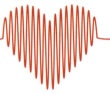

What is an Electrocardiogram

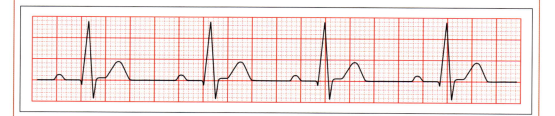

The electrocardiogram, or ECG for short, is defined as the surface recording of the changing voltage generated by the heart as a function of time.

The recording at any given time represents the sum of electrical activity within the entire myocardium.

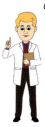

A common mistake is equating electrical activity with contractile activity. There is no information in the ECG about contractility of the heart muscle.

How Electrical Signals Are Detected

Simply applying surface electrodes on the patient and connecting these electrodes via wires to an ECG machine will create the circuit needed for electrocardiographic recordings.

Electrodes pick up electrical activity from the skin. They function as conductors to allow electrical contact with a non metallic part of the circuit which is the patient.

The electrical activity picked up from the electrodes is then transmitted along a cable to the ECG machine where it is amplified and processed. After amplification, the electrical impulse is transformed into mechanical motion. The mechanical action directs the movement of the stylus which forms a tracing on the graphic paper. The paper underneath the stylus moves in order to capture the heart's electrical activity over time.

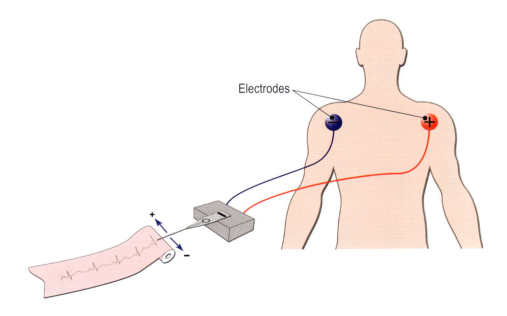

On the graphic paper, the vertical axis represents voltage and the horizontal axis represents time. The stylus only moves (up or down) when voltage is detected. The old stylus paper writing process has been replaced by sophisticated recording systems involving computers.

Brief History of the Electrocardiogram

The first electrical activity from the intact human heart was recorded with a mercury capillary electrometer by Augustus Waller in May 1887 at St. Mary's Hospital, London. The tracings were poor and exhibited only 2 distorted deflections. Willem Einthoven (1860 – 1927) who was professor of physiology at the University of Leiden, The Netherlands, improved the distortion of the ECG with the mercury capillary electrometer but the recordings were still suboptimal. During the early years, working with the mercury capillary electrometer, Einthoven introduced the PQRST designation for the several electrocardiographic deflections as it is known today.

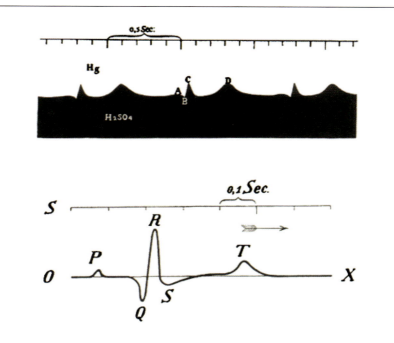

Top: Improved recording of the ECG by Einthoven with the modified capillary electrometer. **Bottom**: The lower tracing is the reconstructed ECG corrected mathematically.

Einthoven eventually improved ECG recordings with the introduction of a very sensitive string galvanometer (an instrument for detecting and measuring small electric current) of his design. He published the first practical ECG in 1902. The Nobel Prize in Physiology or Medicine 1924 was awarded to Willem Einthoven "for his discovery of the mechanism of the electrocardiogram".

The original apparatus in Leiden was huge in size as it filled 2 rooms, weighed 600 pounds, and required 5 people to operate it. Yet, it worked. The clinical use of Einthoven's immobile equipment required transtelephonic transmission of the ECG from the physiology laboratory to the clinic at the Academic Hospital about a mile away.

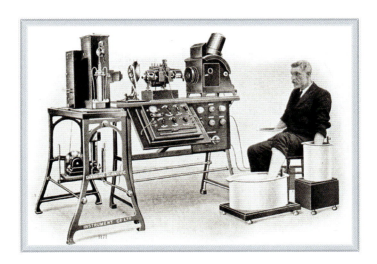

Large buckets of saline were used as electrodes with the subject immersing his hands and feet. The original cylinders of electrolyte solutions were reduced in size and still in use as late as 1930.

While the three-lead electrocardiogram of Einthoven was a satisfactory method to assess arrhythmias, it was soon recognized that there were 'silent areas' in the heart where a myocardial infarction might not be detected. The superior diagnostic yield of a 12-lead ECG was established in the early 1940's based on the work of Frank Wilson of the University of Michigan and Emanuel Goldberger of Lincoln Hospital, New York. This lead arrangement has persisted until now in the form of the standard 12-lead ECG.

Dipole Theory

The heart can be thought of as a dipole. A dipole is the electrical polarity between two points. In other words, it is two charged objects, with equal but opposite charges that are separated by a distance. So, one is positive and the other is negative.

As the cardiac impulse "sweeps" across the heart, there will be some of the myocardium that is electrically active and some that is at rest. This results in a charge separation or dipole.

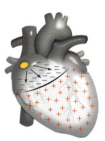

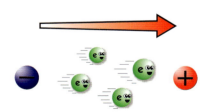

Electrons flow from the negative pole (depolarized areas) of the dipole to the positive pole (polarized areas) which creates an electric field which can be measured in the form of voltage (electrical potential difference) by electrodes.

Note: conventional current assumes that electrons flow from the (+) terminal to the (-) terminal. This was the convention chosen during the discovery of electricity. This was proven incorrect years later after discovery of the electron. Electrons were found to flow from the (-) terminal to the (+) terminal. By the time the electron was discovered, the idea of electricity flowing from (+) to (-) was firmly established and continues to be taught today. This may lead to confusion in situations expressed in terms of current.

Vectors

Vector analysis is a mathematical concept used to represent voltage and helps explain the waveforms seen on the ECG. The "**voltage vector**" of a source always points from its negative pole (tail) to its positive pole (head) which is the direction that electrons flow in the body. The length of the vector represents the amplitude of the voltage.

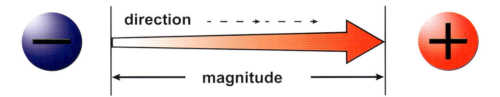

Voltage Vector

Waveform Deflections

This illustration shows the waveform deflections that result from a section of cardiac muscle as it goes through its resting and activated states.

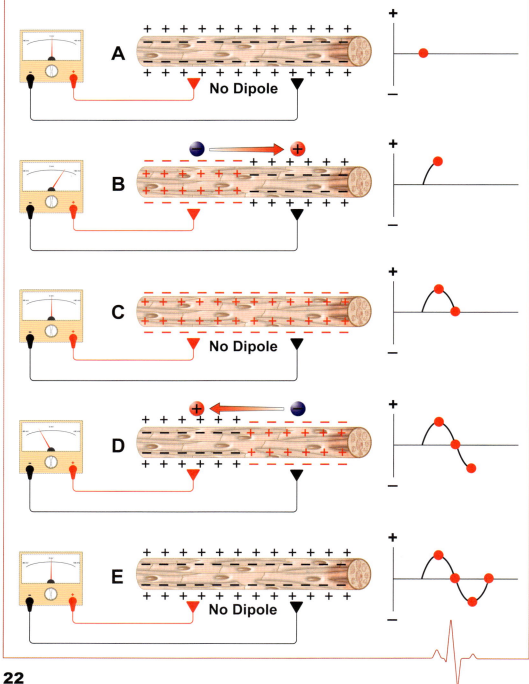

A - Cardiac muscle in its resting state (the charge on the outside of the cells are positive) = no dipole = no voltage vector = no deflection.

B - As the depolarization "wave" sweeps across the muscle, there will be a portion of the muscle that is electrically active (depolarized) with negative charges on the outside of the cells and another portion that has not become electrically active (resting or "polarized" state) with positive charges on the outside of the cells. This is represented by the following voltage vector and produces a positive deflection.

C - Eventually, the entire muscle becomes electrically active (depolarized) = no dipole = no voltage vector = no deflection.

D - The first part of the muscle then returns back to its resting state (repolarization) in the opposite direction. This generates a voltage vector in the opposite direction resulting in a negative deflection.

E - Eventually, the entire muscle returns back to its resting state = no dipole = no voltage vector = no deflection.

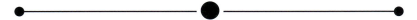

The ECG is simply the registration of the projection of the heart's voltage vector upon what we call the lead axis.

A **lead** refers to a particular combination of two electrodes and the **lead axis** refers to the hypothetical line between these two electrodes. Any pair of electrodes, one (-) and one (+), is used to measure the electrical potential difference (voltage) between two points.

One example of a lead used in electrocardiography is lead I. The (-) electrode is over the right arm and the (+) electrode is over the left arm.

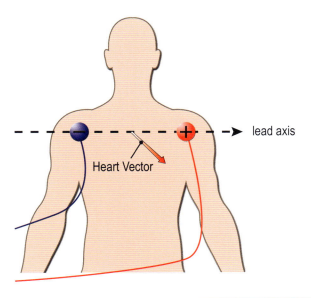

The direction of the deflection (up or down) depends upon which pole (positive or negative) the voltage vector is pointing towards on the lead axis. The deflection on the ECG will be positive if the projection of the voltage vector points to the positive pole of the lead axis and negative if it points to the negative pole of the lead axis.

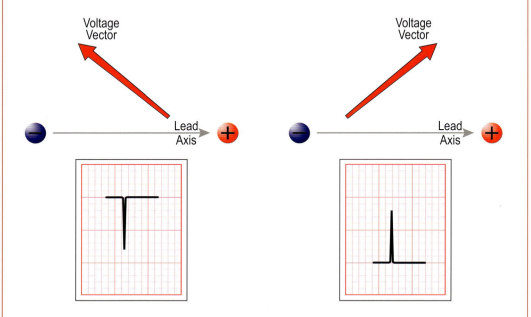

The magnitude of the deflection on the ECG is determined by the angle between the voltage vector and the lead axis. The smaller the angle, the greater the magnitude. A vector that is perpendicular to the lead axis will show no deflection at all.

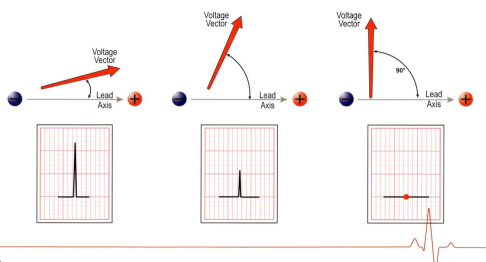

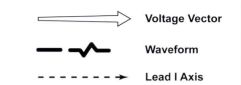
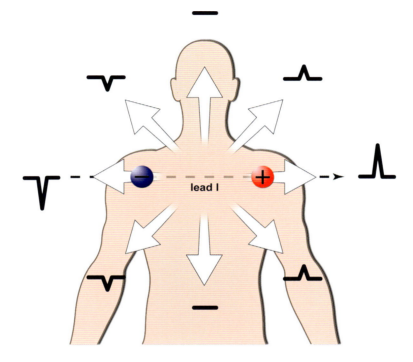

The voltage vector is continuously changing as the heart undergoes electrical activation so the deflections will vary over time.

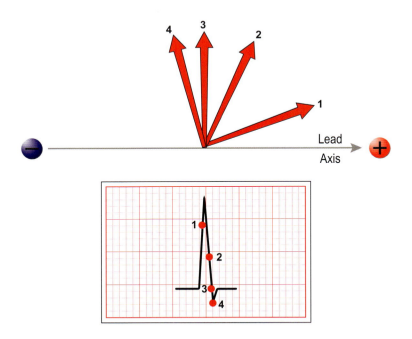

Since the heart is three dimensional, the voltage vector and lead axis need to be represented in 3D as well. Here we introduce three dimensionality to the perpendicular plane of this particular lead so any heart vector that falls to the left of this plane will be negative and to the right will be positive.

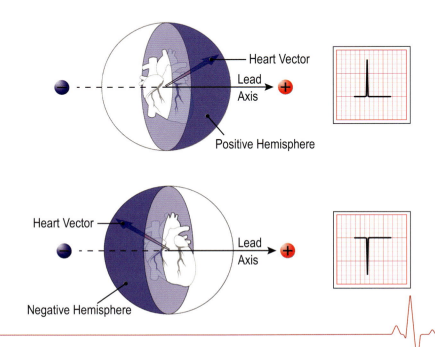

ECG Leads

12 Different Viewpoints

In electrocardiography, there are 12 different leads (electrode combinations) available. Each lead captures a different "point of view" of the heart allowing the 12-lead ECG to capture the electrical behavior of many different areas of the heart simultaneously.

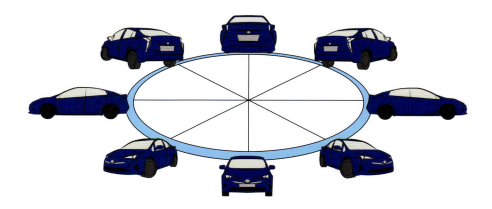

Leads may be divided into two groups based on anatomical orientation.

Frontal Plane Leads **Transverse (Horizontal) Plane Leads**

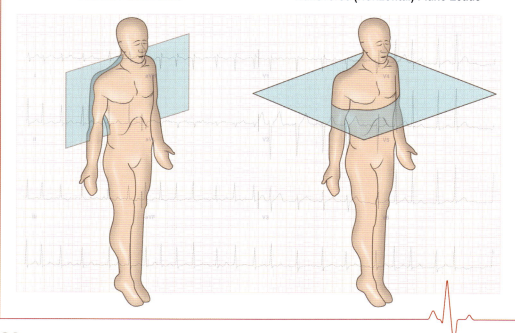

Frontal Plane Lead Systems

Frontal Plane Orientation of the Heart

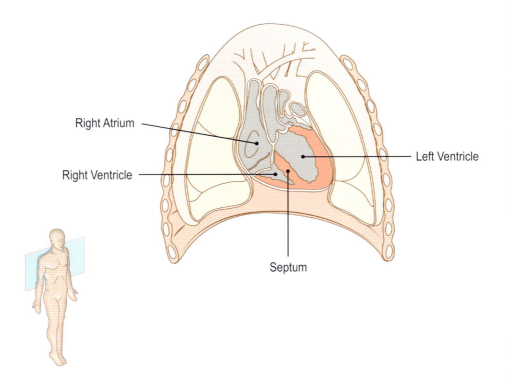

There are two frontal plane lead systems:

1 Standard Limb leads (Bipolar): I, II and III

2 Augmented leads (Unipolar): aVR, aVL and aVF

Standard Limb Leads (I, II and III)

I, II and III are considered **bipolar** leads. Bipolar leads have exploring electrodes on two different parts of the body.

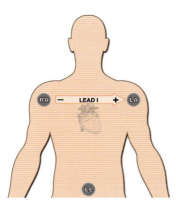

Lead I has the (-) electrode on the right arm (RA) and the (+) electrode on the left arm (LA)

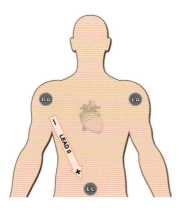

Lead II has the (-) electrode on the right arm and the (+) electrode on the left leg (LL)

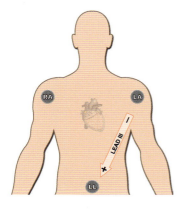

Lead III has the (-) electrode on the left arm and the (+) electrode on the left leg

The limb leads were the first to be discovered by Einthoven back in 1902. Einthoven also conceived the famous equilateral triangle with leads I, II, and III at its sides which later became known as **Einthoven's Triangle**.

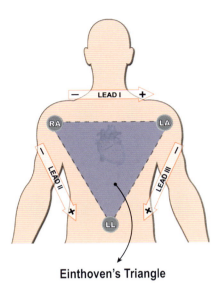

Einthoven's Triangle

He also formulated that lead II - lead I = lead III. This later became known as **Einthoven's Law**.

$$\text{Lead I} + \text{Lead III} - \text{Lead II} = 0$$

The ECG machine assigns the charge, positive or negative, to the electrode and is able to switch back and forth depending on which lead is being investigated.

Augmented Leads (aVR, aVL and aVF)

aVR, aVL and aVF are **unipolar** leads. Unipolar leads have just one exploring (+) electrode on the body. Actually, unipolar leads are bipolar leads because the connecting electrode is at zero potential. The exploring (+) electrode is physically on the body and the (-) electrode (or zero electrode) is an artificially constructed reference called the Wilson's Central Terminal (WCT). It is the simple average of the three exploring electrodes connected to the right arm (RA), left arm (LA) and left leg (LL) and assumed to be steady and of negligible amplitude during the cardiac cycle.

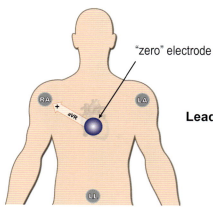

Lead aVR has the (+) electrode on the right arm

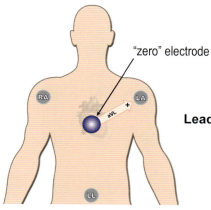

Lead aVL has the (+) electrode on the left arm

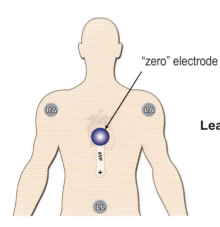

Lead aVF has the (+) electrode on the left leg.

The "a" before the unipolar limb leads (VL, VR and VF) stands for "augmented". The original unipolar limb leads produced waveforms that were too small in amplitude. Modification of the electrode arrangement resulted in a 50% augmentation of the waveform amplitude produced by these unipolar leads.

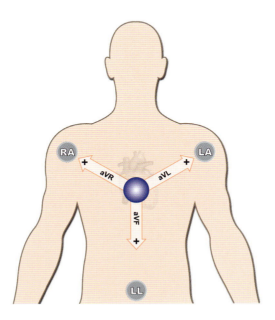

Frontal Plane Hexaxial Diagram

The relationship between the six frontal leads (I, II, III, aVR, aVL and aVF) and the area of the heart they "see" can be more easily understood by using the hexaxial diagram.

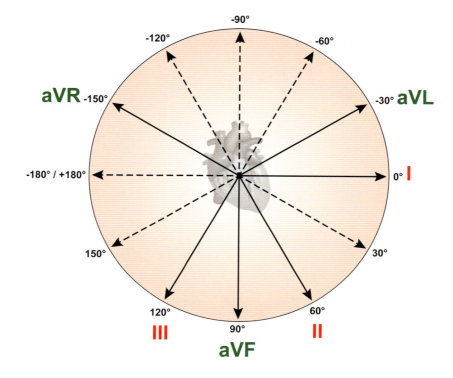

In physics, the projection of a vector on to a particular axis remains the same when the axis is shifted in parallel to its original direction.

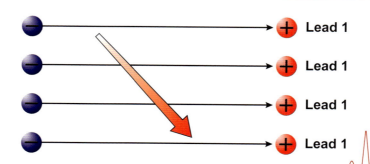

Using this principle, all of the limb lead axises can be shifted in parallel so that they all intersect the electrical center of the heart.

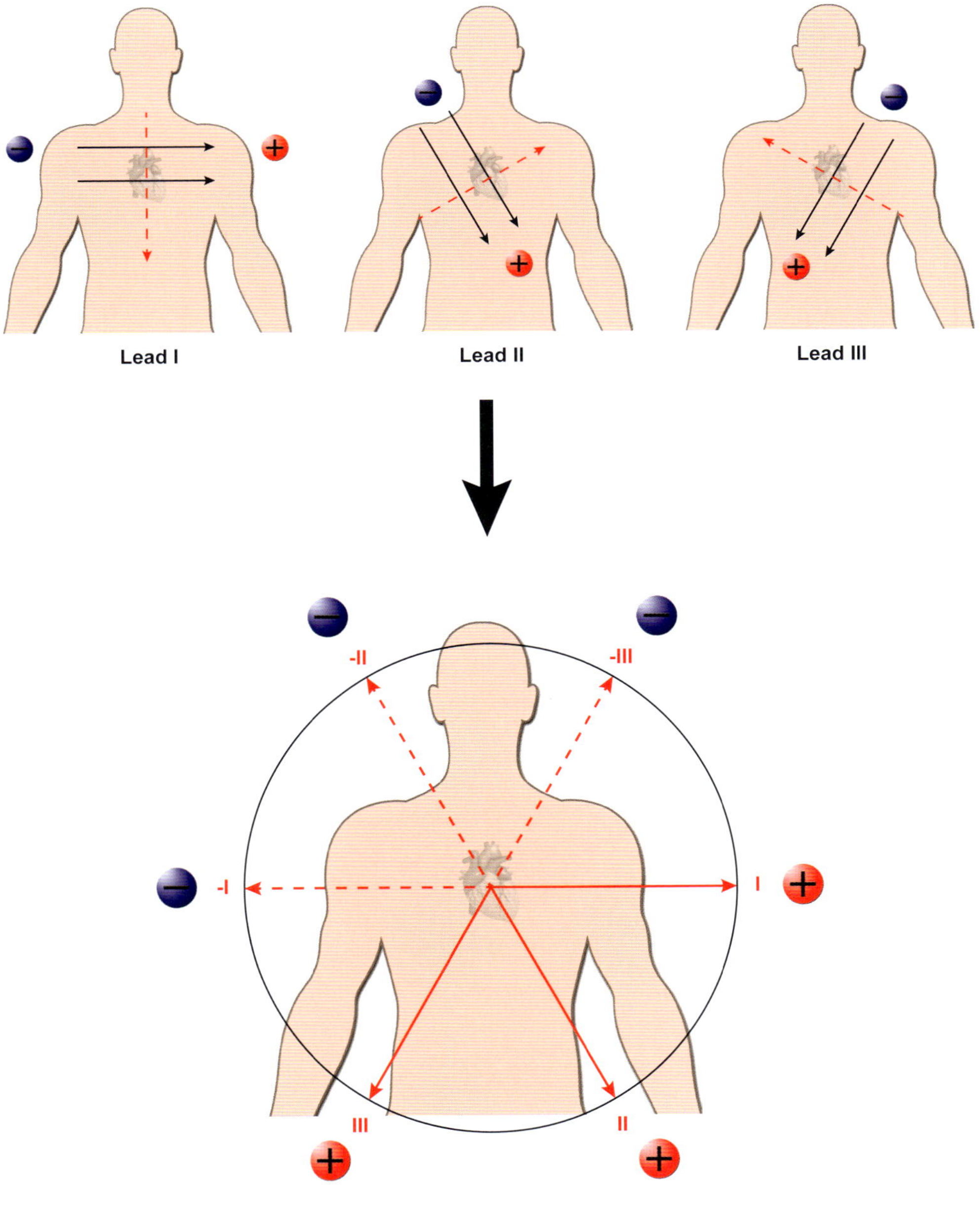
Lead I
Lead II
Lead III
-II
-III
-I
I
III
II

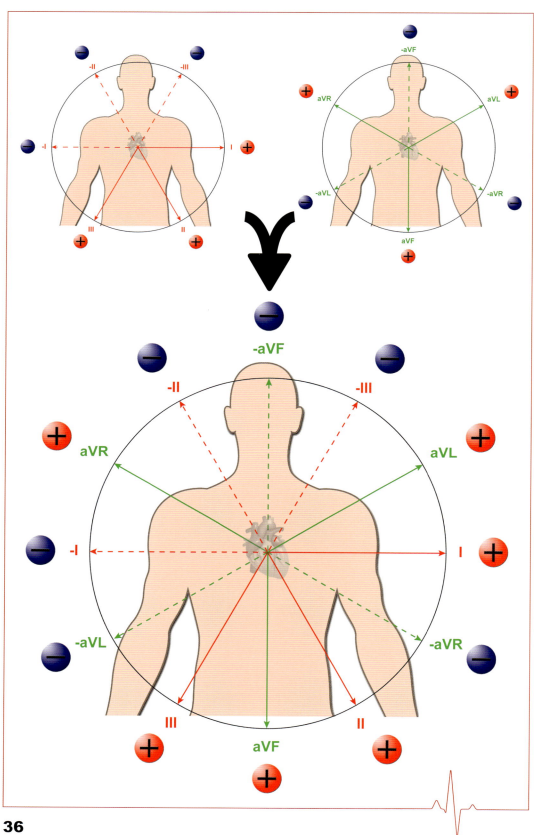

36

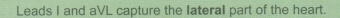

Leads I and aVL capture the **lateral** part of the heart.

Leads II, III and aVF capture the **inferior** part of the heart.

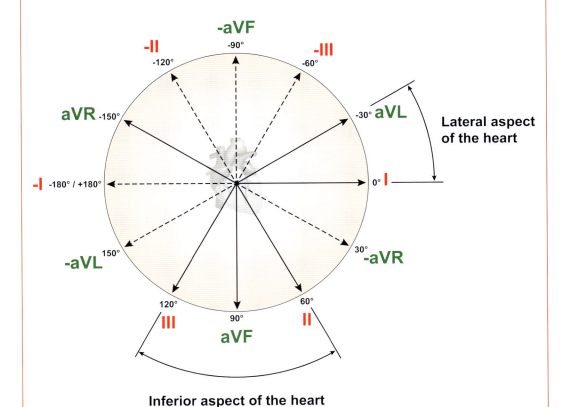

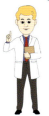

The hexaxial frontal plane diagram is the key to understanding the relationships of the various frontal plane leads.

Transverse Plane Lead System

Transverse Plane Orientation of the Heart

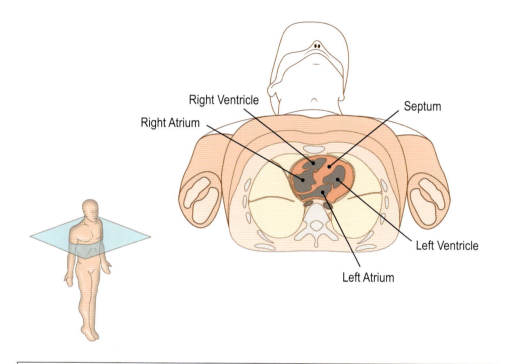

The transverse plane lead system:

 Precordial or Chest Leads (Unipolar):
V1, V2, V3, V4, V5 and V6

All of the precordial leads are **unipolar** leads because the electrical potential difference is between the "zero" electrode and an exploring electrode located over a particular area on the chest wall.

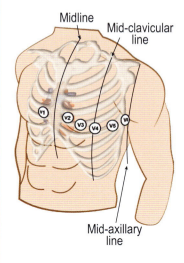

The normal position of the (+) electrodes

V1 - right side of the sternum in the fourth intercostal space

V2 - left side of the sternum in the fourth intercostal space

V3 - midway between V2 and V4

V4 - mid-clavicular line in the fifth intercostal space

V5 - anterior axillary line at the same level as V4

V6 - mid-axillary line at the same level as V4

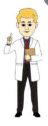

Proper positioning of the precordial electrodes is very important. Misplacement can result in diagnostic errors.

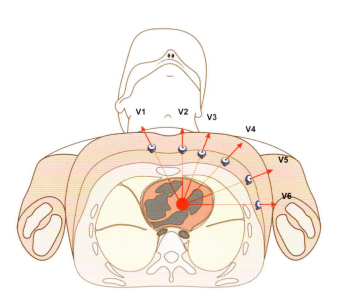

Leads V1 and V2 capture the **septum** of the heart.

Leads V3 and V4 capture the **anterior** part of the heart.

Leads V5 and V6 capture the **lateral** part of the heart.

Views of the Heart & Corresponding Leads

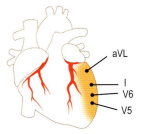

Leads I, aVL, V5 and V6 capture the **lateral** part of the heart

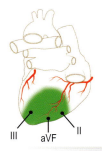

Leads II, III and aVF capture the **inferior** part of the heart

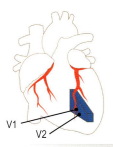

Leads V1 and V2 capture the **septum**

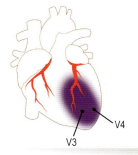

Leads V3 and V4 capture the **anterior** part of the heart

12-Lead ECG Format

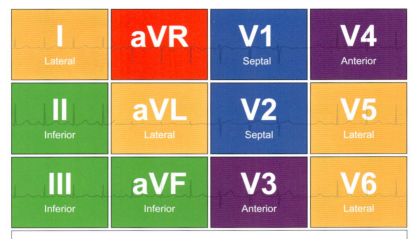

12-Lead ECG Recording Procedure

For a comprehensive 12-lead ECG recording, the procedure involves placing electrodes at 10 anatomical locations on the surface of the body. The electrode placed over the right leg (RL) is the ground and not included in any recordings.

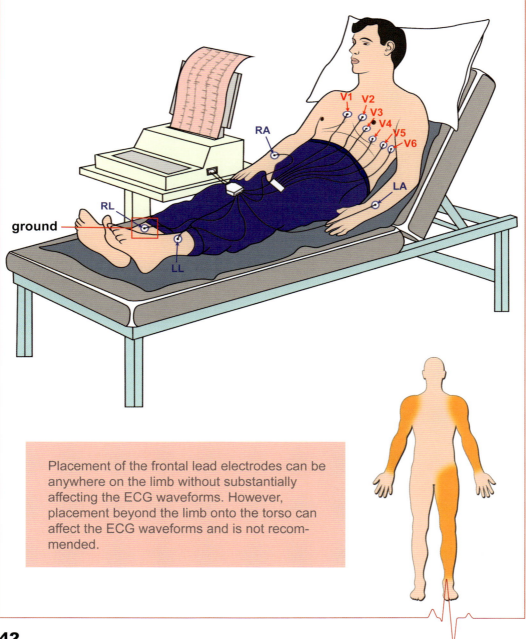

Placement of the frontal lead electrodes can be anywhere on the limb without substantially affecting the ECG waveforms. However, placement beyond the limb onto the torso can affect the ECG waveforms and is not recommended.

42

ECG Waveforms, Axis and Intervals

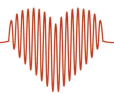

ECG Paper

The paper on which the ECG is recorded is preprinted with horizontal lines representing time and vertical lines representing voltage amplitude.

The standard ECG is recorded at a paper speed of 25 mm/second and a gain setting (calibration) of 10 mm/mV (millivolt). All interpretations by waveform measurements are based on these standards.

A calibration of 10 mm/mV means that a 1 mV signal produces a 10 mm deflection on the ECG grid. It is important to check that it is calibrated correctly. Calibration signals are marked at the start of the recording.

Each **large square** is measured to be 5.0 mm = 0.5 mV on the vertical axis and 0.20 seconds on the horizontal axis.

Each large square is made up of 5 small squares measured to be 1.0 mm = 0.1 mV on the vertical axis and 0.04 seconds on the horizontal axis.

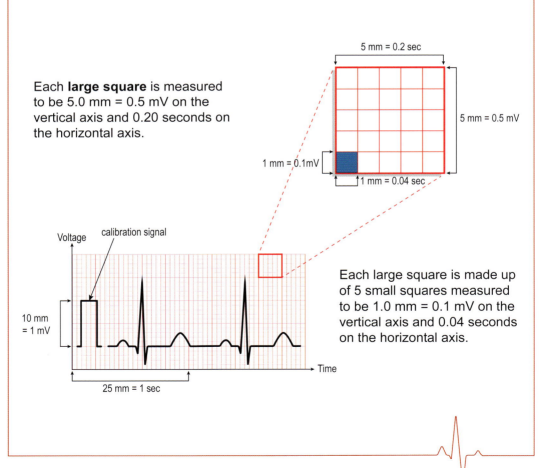

44

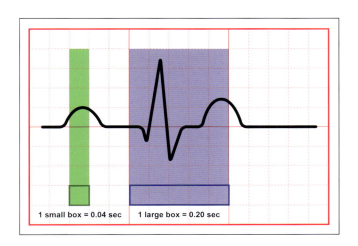

Measuring Time

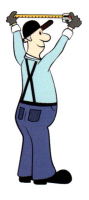
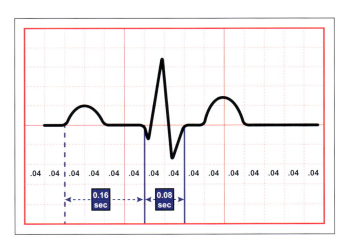

Measuring Voltage

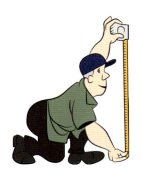
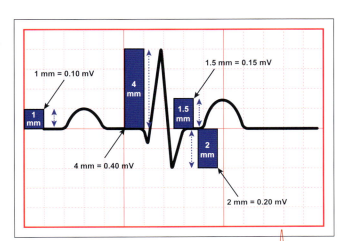

45

Isoelectric Line

All measurements of voltage on the ECG are relative to the ECG isoelectric line where there is no measurable voltage. A deflection above the isoelectric line is called "positive" and a deflection below is called "negative".

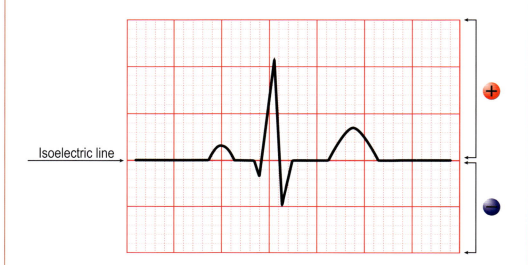

ECG Waveforms

There are **three** distinct waveforms in a normal ECG cycle:
1) **P wave** which represents electrical activation (depolarization) of the atria.
2) **QRS complex** which represents electrical activation (depolarization) of the ventricles.
3) **T wave** which represents recovery (repolarization) of the ventricles.

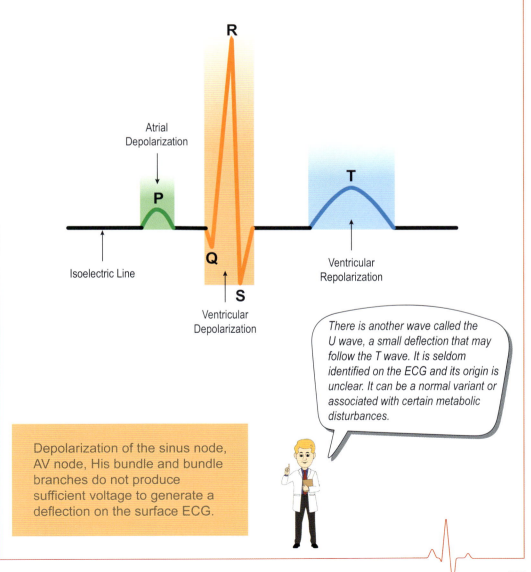

Depolarization of the sinus node, AV node, His bundle and bundle branches do not produce sufficient voltage to generate a deflection on the surface ECG.

There is another wave called the U wave, a small deflection that may follow the T wave. It is seldom identified on the ECG and its origin is unclear. It can be a normal variant or associated with certain metabolic disturbances.

P Wave

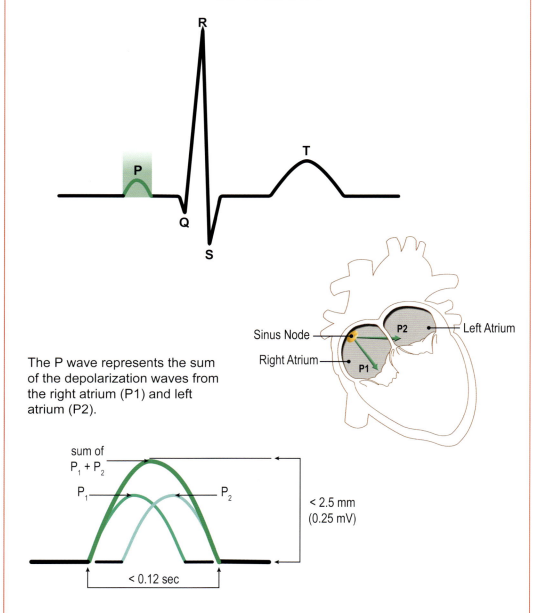

The P wave represents the sum of the depolarization waves from the right atrium (P1) and left atrium (P2).

The normal P wave has a smooth contour, is not normally peaked or pointed, is **< 0.12 sec** (3 small boxes) and does not exceed an amplitude of **2.5 mm** (2½ small boxes) in the frontal leads. The ECG reflects that atrial depolarization occurs from top to bottom.

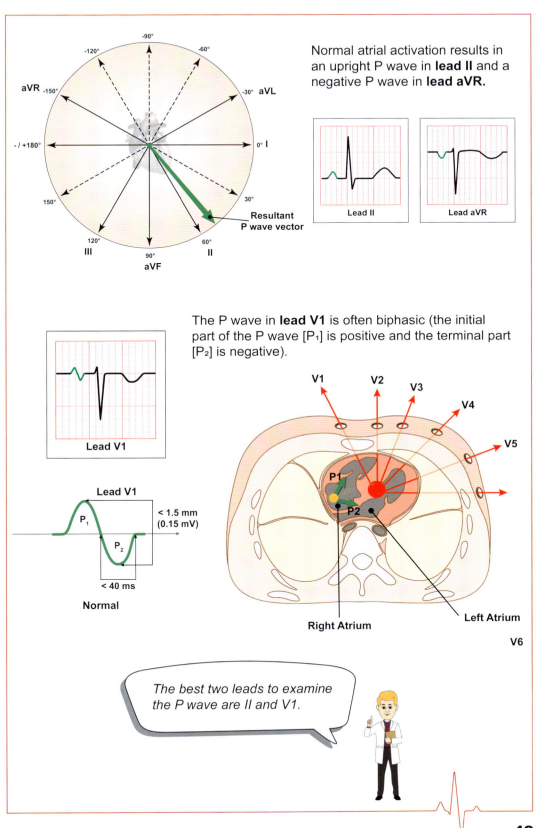

QRS Complex

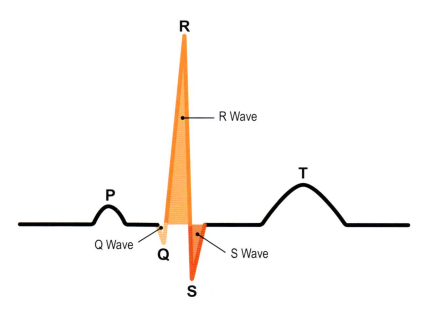

The **QRS complex** represents ventricular activation and may be comprised of one or more deflections. As a general rule, if the first deflection is negative, it is called a **Q wave**. An **R wave** is the first positive deflection which may or may not be preceded by a Q wave. Any negative deflection preceded by an upward deflection (R wave) is called an **S wave**.

Any arrangement reflecting ventricular activation is called a "QRS" complex even though one or more of these deflections (Q,R,S) may be absent.

Although there can only be one Q wave in a QRS complex, there may be more than one R or S wave. Any second positive deflection is indicated by an accent (R' = R prime or S' = S prime). An upper case letter (Q, R, S, QS) is assigned to the large waves that form the major deflections and a lower case (q, r, s) is assigned to the smaller waves that are less than 1/2 the amplitude of the larger deflection. A single large Q wave with no positive deflection is labeled a QS complex.

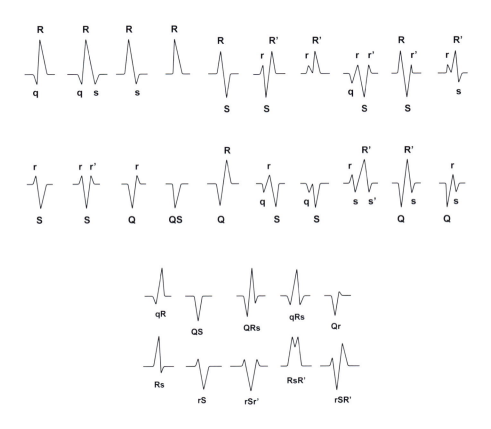

Origin of the QRS Complex

The **initial heart vector** (HV$_I$) is directed from left to right as the impulse is conducted down the left and right bundle branches. During this initial phase, depolarization involves the ventricular septum.

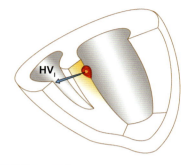

The second heart vector, referred to as the "**main**" **heart vector** (HV$_M$), is directed to the left, posteriorly and inferiorly. During this phase, depolarization mainly involves the anterolateral and posterolateral regions of the heart

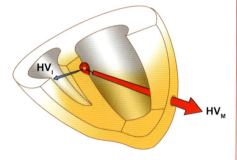

The third or **terminal heart vector** (HV$_T$) is directed backwards, upwards and either left or right. It represents depolarization of the basal regions of the heart.

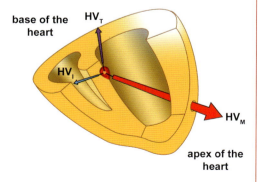

The appearance of the QRS complex depends on which lead is being recorded. Normally, small q waves are visible in the anterolateral leads (I, aVL, V5 and V6) as a result of septal depolarization.

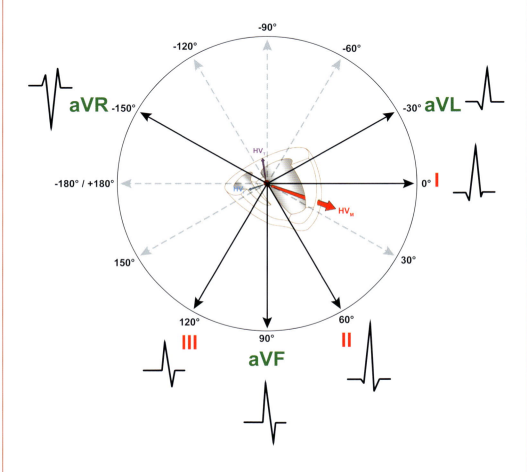

With the precordial leads, the R wave amplitude normally increases and the S wave amplitude normally decreases when moving from lead V1 (right side of heart) to lead V6 (left lateral part of the heart).

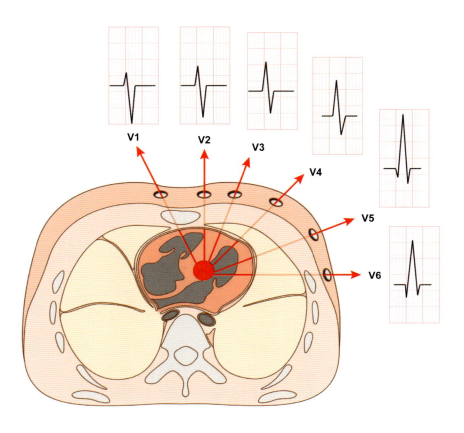

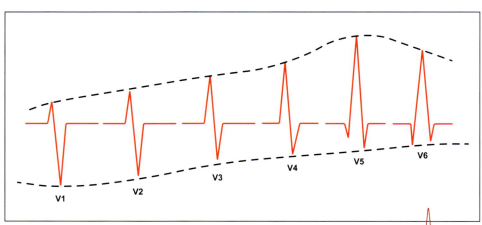

QRS Width

The width of the QRS complex represents the intraventricular conduction time, the time it takes for the ventricles to become completely depolarized. The normal QRS duration is 0.06 - 0.10 seconds (1½ - 2½ small boxes) and is measured from the start of the first QRS deflection to the end of the last QRS deflection. A prolonged QRS complex of > 0.10 seconds, referred to as a "wide" QRS, indicates an intraventricular conduction disturbance.

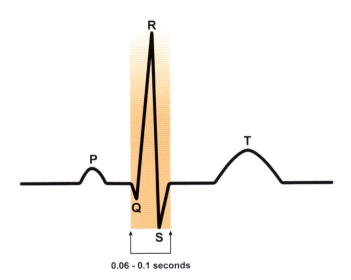

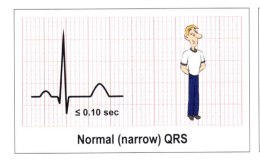

Normal (narrow) QRS

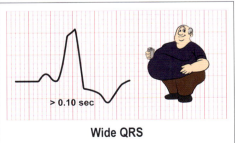

Wide QRS

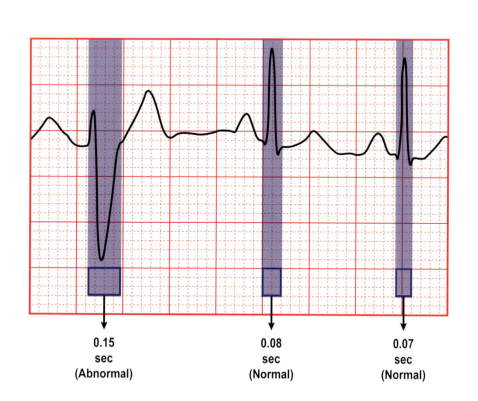

0.15 sec (Abnormal)   0.08 sec (Normal)   0.07 sec (Normal)

QRS Axis

The mean **QRS axis** is the net overall direction of electrical activity in the frontal plane and within a normal heart it falls between +90° and -30° (left and inferior). An axis that falls outside of this range is considered abnormal.

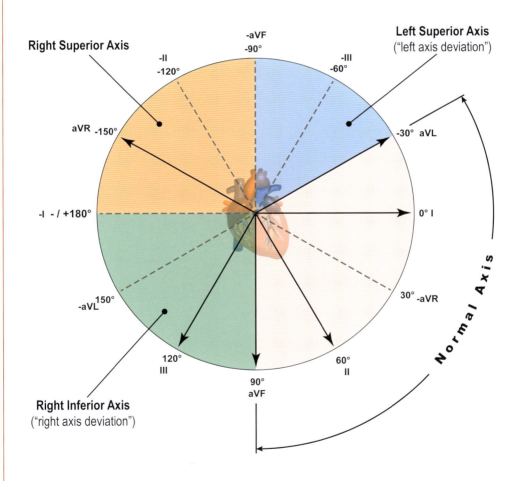

The fastest way to determine the mean QRS axis involves comparing the QRS complex in **lead I** and **lead aVF**.

Determine the main QRS direction (positive or negative) in lead I and aVF.

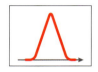 or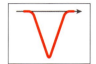

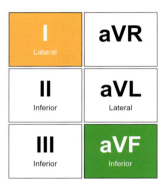

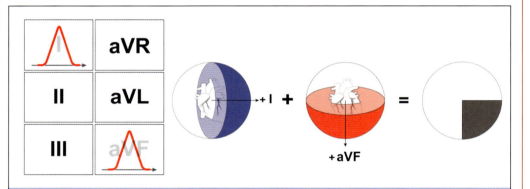

If both leads are positive, the axis is within the normal range.

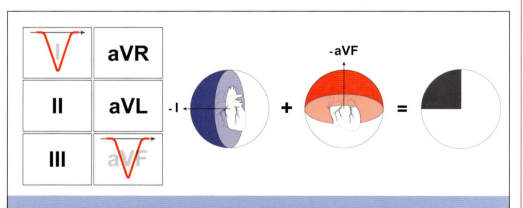

If both leads are negative, there is a right superior axis.

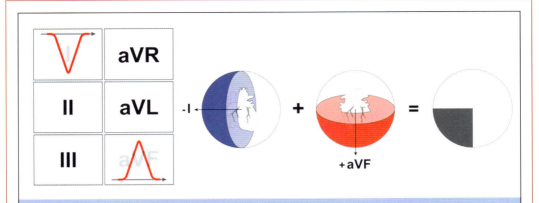

If lead I is negative and lead aVF is positive, there is a right inferior axis (right axis deviation).

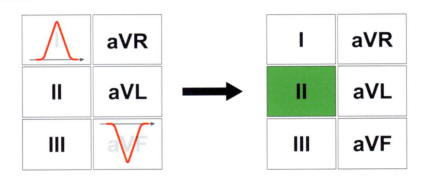

If lead I is positive and lead aVF negative, the axis may be normal or abnormal. Looking at lead II will provide the answer if normal (up to -30°) or not (-30 to -90°).

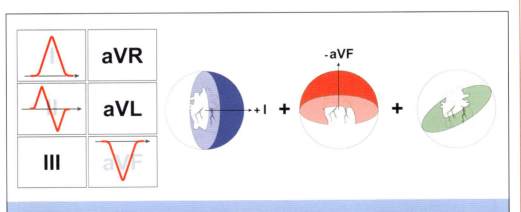

If Lead II is equiphasic (positive and negative forces cancel each other), the axis is directed along lead aVL at -30°.

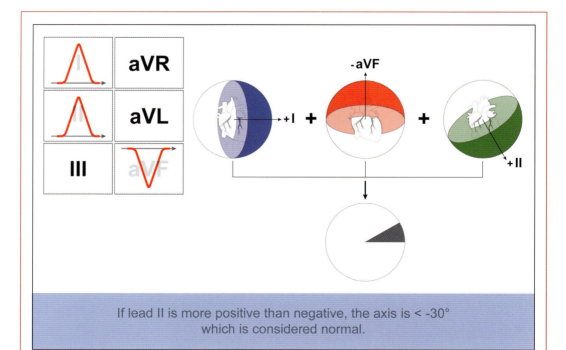

If lead II is more positive than negative, the axis is < -30° which is considered normal.

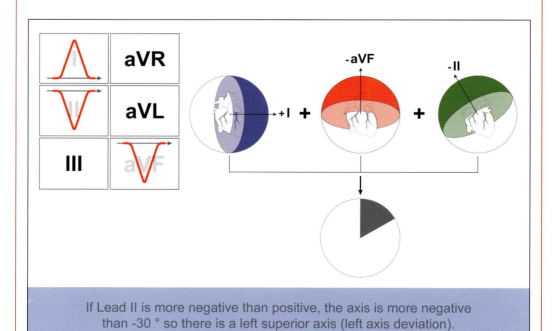

If Lead II is more negative than positive, the axis is more negative than -30 ° so there is a left superior axis (left axis deviation).

T Wave

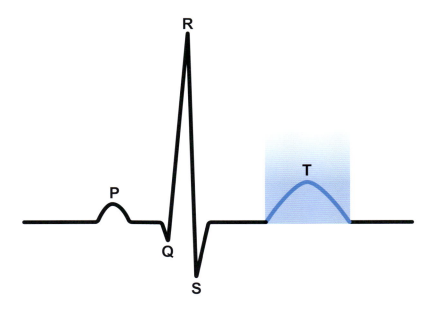

The **T wave** is the most variable wave on the ECG. The T wave provides visible evidence of the repolarization process. The normal T wave is generally in the same direction as the main QRS deflection, is upright in leads I, II, V3 to V6 and always inverted in lead aVR.

Why isn't the T wave in the opposite direction since repolarization is the opposite to depolarization? One would expect that the first area to depolarize would be the first to repolarize but that is not the case in the ventricular wall. Depolarization normally begins in the endocardium (inner layer of the heart) and ends in the epicardium (outer layer of the heart), however, the opposite occurs with repolarization. The endocardium depolarizes first and repolarizes last so the direction of the voltage vector does not change.

Depolarization

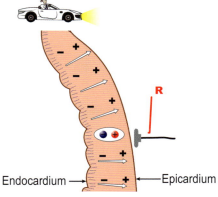

Partial Depolarization

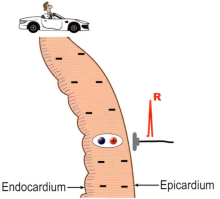

Depolarization Complete

Repolarization

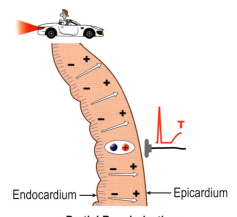

Partial Repolarization

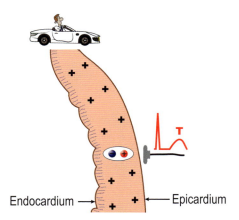

Repolarization Complete

ST Segment

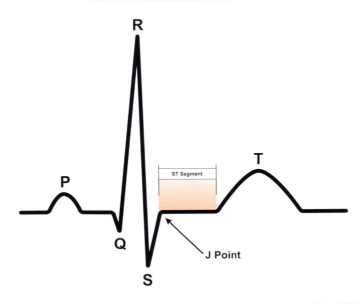

The ST segment is the part of the ECG between the end of the QRS complex and the onset of the T wave. The J point, the junction between the QRS complex and the ST segment, is where the repolarization phase of the ventricles begins. Normally, the ST segment is isoelectric. An ST segment above ("ST Elevation") or below ("ST Depression") the isoelectric line is considered abnormal.

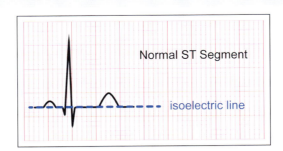

Normal ST Segment

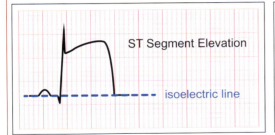

ST Segment Elevation

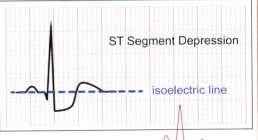

ST Segment Depression

63

ECG Intervals

PR Interval

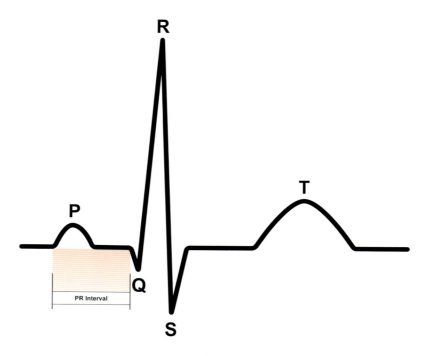

The PR interval is measured from the onset of the P wave to the onset of the QRS complex and represents the time it takes for the impulse to travel from the sinus node through the AV node. The normal PR Interval is 0.12 - 0.20 sec (3-5 small boxes).

QT Interval

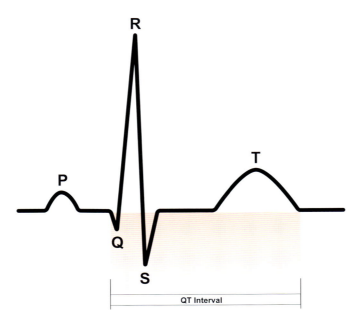

The QT interval is measured from the onset of the QRS complex to the end of the T wave and represents the total time from the onset of ventricular depolarization to complete repolarization. Since the QT interval varies with heart rate, measurements are usually corrected for heart rate (QTc). The normal QTc for women is < 0.46 sec and men is < 0.44 sec.

$$QTc = \frac{QT}{\sqrt{R\text{-}R}}*$$

* the RR interval is described on the next page

RR Interval

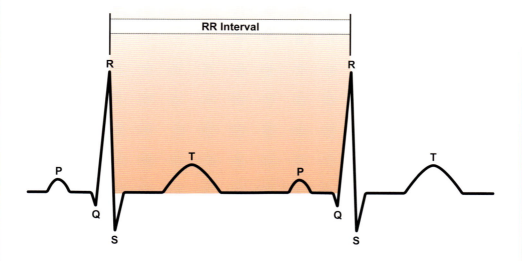

The RR Interval is the measurement between the R wave within one cardiac electrical cycle and the R wave in the next cycle and is used to determine the **regularity** of the rhythm and the **heart rate**.

Comparing the RR intervals over time determines the regularity of a rhythm. If the RR intervals are consistently the same, the rhythm is considered "regular". If they are inconsistent, the rhythm is considered "irregular".

The mathematical analysis of the RR intervals over time determines the heart rate. Heart rate, expressed as beats per minute (bpm), can be calculated a few different ways when the rhythm is regular.

Methods of Determining Heart Rate:

1. The 300 Method
2. The 1500 Method
3. Cardiac Ruler Method
4. 6 Second Method

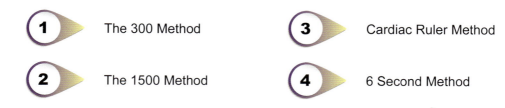

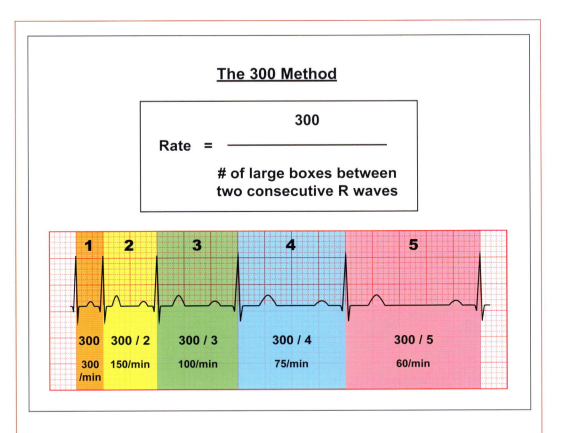

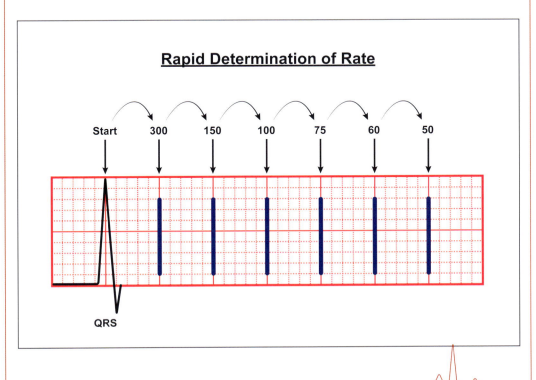

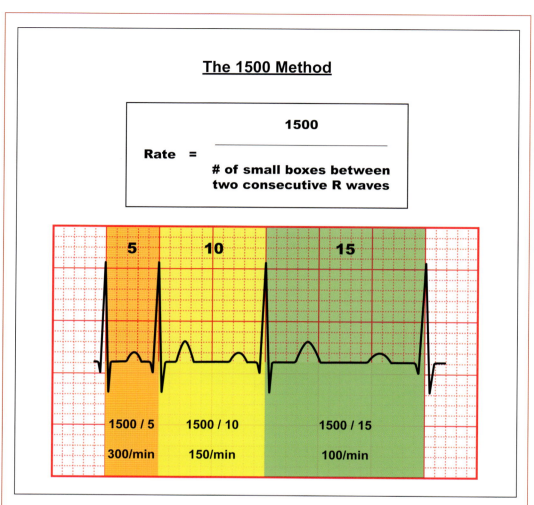

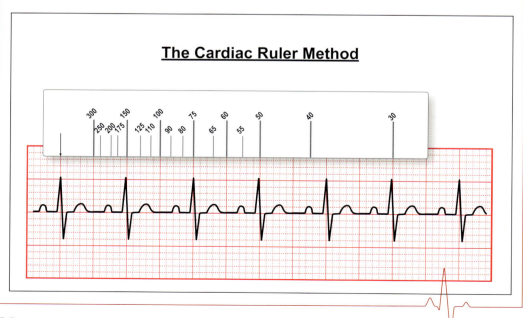

The Six Second Method

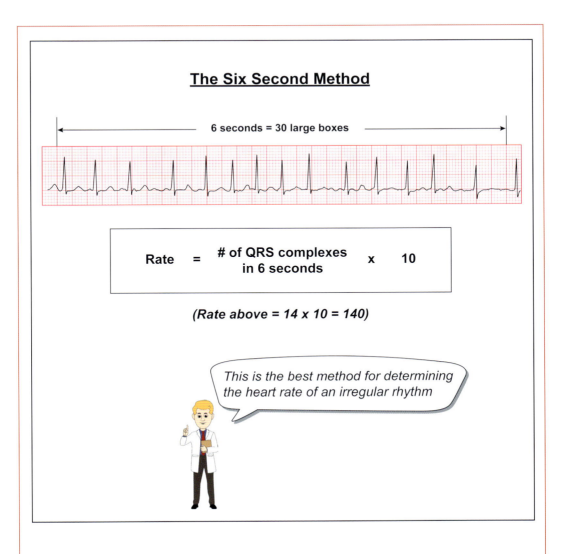

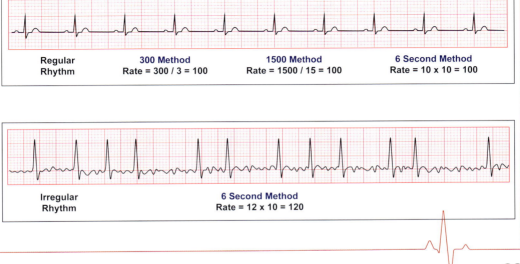

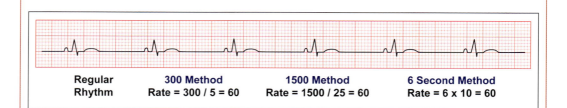

Regular Rhythm | 300 Method Rate = 300 / 5 = 60 | 1500 Method Rate = 1500 / 25 = 60 | 6 Second Method Rate = 6 x 10 = 60

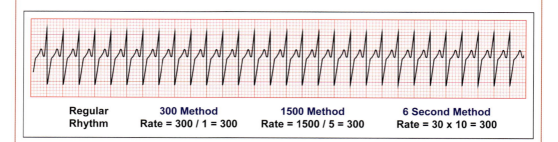

Regular Rhythm | 300 Method Rate = 300 / 1 = 300 | 1500 Method Rate = 1500 / 5 = 300 | 6 Second Method Rate = 30 x 10 = 300

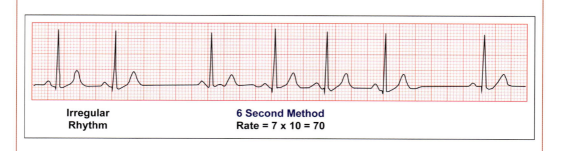

Irregular Rhythm | 6 Second Method Rate = 7 x 10 = 70

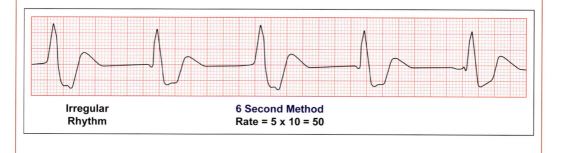

Irregular Rhythm | 6 Second Method Rate = 5 x 10 = 50

PP Interval

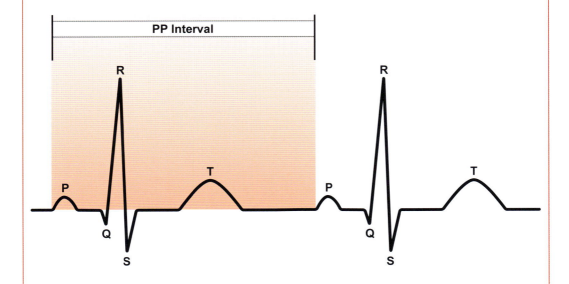

The PP Interval is the interval between P waves and is measured from the onset of one P wave to the onset of the next P wave. The mathematical analysis of the PP intervals over time determines the atrial rate. The methods used to calculate the ventricular rate can also be used to calculate the atrial rate. This calculation can be valuable when evaluating for certain rhythm disturbances.

Sinus Rhythm

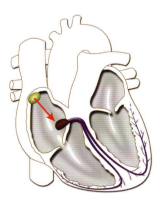

The normal rhythm of the heart originates in the SA node. **Sinus rhythm** is a term used to describe atrial activation by an impulse traveling from the sinoatrial (SA) node to the AV node. Because the SA node does not produce sufficient voltage to produce a deflection on the surface ECG, its behavior is inferred from the appearance of the P wave.

Upright or positive P waves in lead II and inverted or negative P waves in lead aVR reflect the normal superior to inferior activation sequence of the atria.

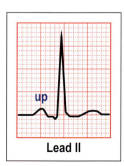

Lead II

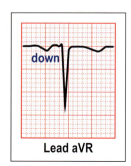

Lead aVR

The term "normal" sinus rhythm (NSR) is used to describe a regular sinus rhythm with a rate between 60 and 100/min <u>regardless</u> of the status of AV conduction.

Sinus bradycardia refers to a sinus rhythm with a HR < 60/min. Sinus tachycardia refers to a sinus rhythm with a HR > 100/min.

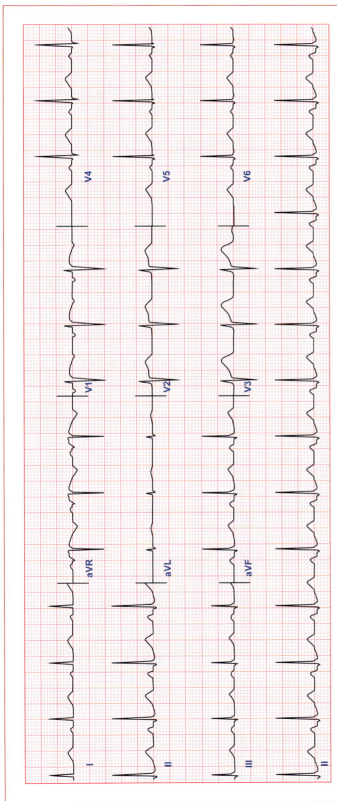

The P waves are upright in lead II and negative in lead aVR and the heart rate is 83 indicating a normal sinus rhythm. The mean frontal plan QRS axis is normal. The PR intervals are constant and normal. There is 1:1 AV conduction.

Normal ECG Measurements

P wave	smooth contour, < 0.12 sec, < 2.5 mm, upright in lead II and inverted in lead aVR
QRS duration	≤ 0.10 sec
R wave progression	R wave amplitude increases and S wave decreases from V1 to V6
QRS Axis	axis between -30° to 90°
T wave	generally the same direction as the main QRS deflection, upright in leads I, II, V3 to V6 and always inverted in lead aVR
ST segment	isoelectric (without elevation or depression)
PR interval	0.12 - 0.20 sec
QTc interval	< 0.46 sec (women) & < 0.44 sec (men)
Heart rate (resting)	60 - 100/min, although 50 is considered normal for some individuals (i.e. athletes)
Rhythm	sinus, no variations in PR intervals, RR intervals are regular and the P waves precede the QRS complexes in a ratio of 1:1

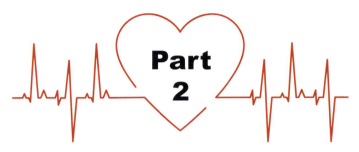

Specific Morphological Abnormalities

Atrial Abnormalities

The term "atrial abnormality" has replaced the previous commonly used term "atrial enlargement" because atrial hypertrophy (thickened wall), atrial conduction delay and atrial dilatation (enlargement) can all produce the same abnormal ECG pattern.

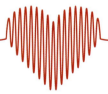

Left Atrial Abnormality

The characteristic ECG patterns of left atrial abnormality include:

 A broad (> 0.12 sec) and notched P wave best seen in **lead II**.

 Deeply inverted or negative second part of the P wave in **lead V1**.

	Normal P Wave	Left Atrial Abnormality
LEAD II	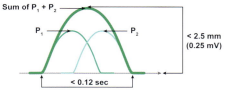 Normal	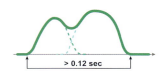 Broad and Notched P wave
LEAD V1	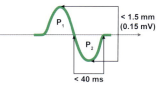 Normal	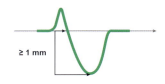 Deeply inverted P$_2$

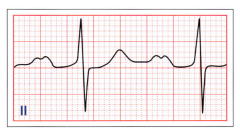
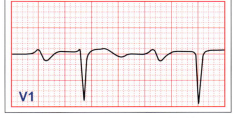

Sinus rhythm with left atrial abnormality. The P wave in lead II is broad (0.16 sec) and notched. Lead V1 shows a predominantly negative (inverted) terminal P wave.

Right Atrial Abnormality

The characteristic ECG patterns of right atrial abnormality include:

 The P wave has a high amplitude (> 2.5 mm in leads II, III and aVF and > 1.5 mm in leads V1 and V2).

Normal P Wave / Right Atrial Abnormality

LEAD II — Normal (Sum of $P_1 + P_2$, < 2.5 mm (0.25 mV), < 0.12 sec) / High Amplitude P Wave (> 2.5 mm (0.25 mV))

LEAD V1 — Normal (> 1.5 mm (0.15 mV), < 40 ms) / High Amplitude P Wave (> 0.15 mV)

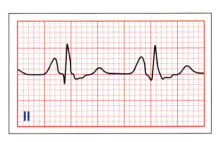

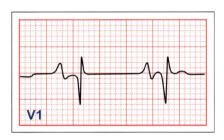

Sinus rhythm with right atrial abnormality. Note the high amplitude P wave present in both lead II and V1.

Ventricular Hypertrophy

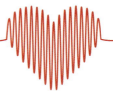

Left Ventricular Hypertrophy

Ventricular hypertrophy is defined as thickening of the muscle wall of the ventricle.

Normal Heart **Left Ventricular Hypertrophy**

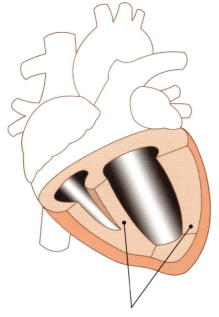 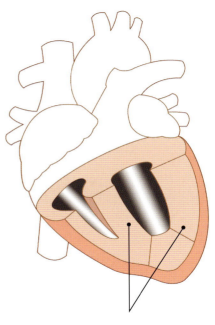

Normal left ventricular wall   Thickened left ventricular wall

The ECG criteria for diagnosing hypertrophy are not very sensitive (the ECG changes are not always present even if the condition is present in the heart) but are very specific (if the ECG changes are present then hypertrophy is likely to be present).

Several diagnostic ECG criteria for left ventricular hypertrophy (LVH) have been used. Here are few common ones:

1 The amplitude of the S wave in leads V1 or V2 plus the amplitude of the R wave in leads V5 or V6 (whichever is larger) is ≥ 35 mm (7 large vertical boxes). This is the most used criterion to diagnose left ventricular hypertrophy.

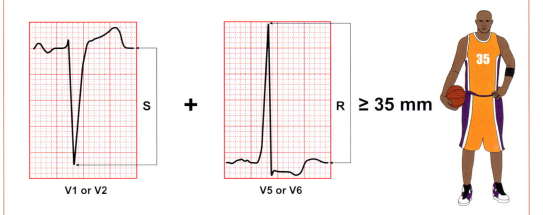

2 Other commonly used criteria include an R wave in lead aVL that is ≥ 11 mm or a delayed intrinsicoid deflection (the time from the beginning of the QRS to the peak of the R wave) in lead V6.

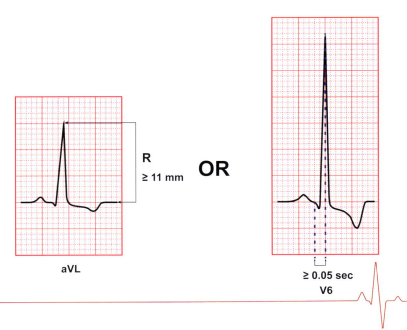

With left ventricular hypertrophy, the ST segments and T waves are usually opposite in direction to the main deflection of the QRS complexes. This is often referred to as a left ventricular strain pattern.

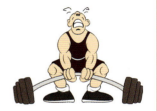

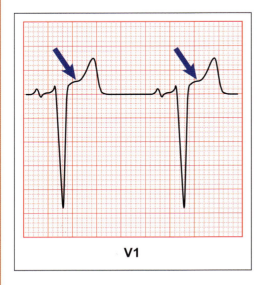

V1

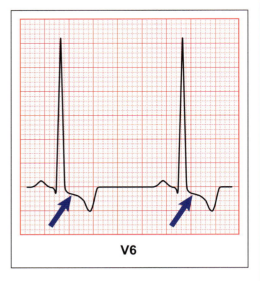

V6

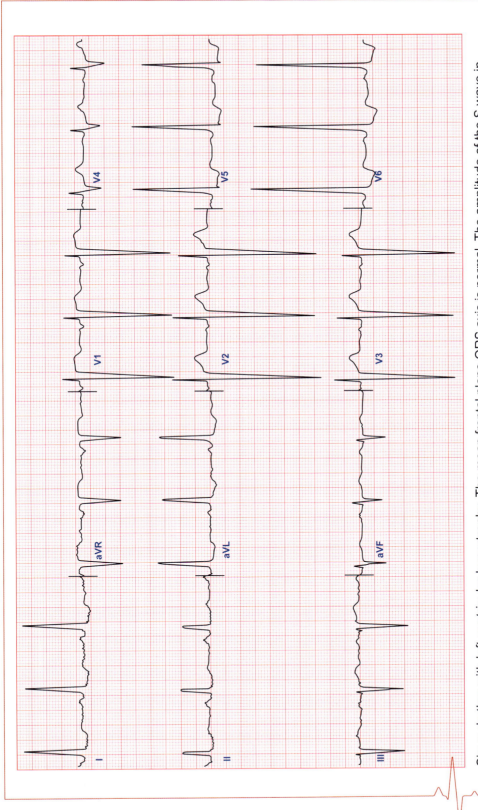

Sinus rhythm with left ventricular hypertrophy. The mean frontal plane QRS axis is normal. The amplitude of the S wave in lead V2 plus the R wave in lead V6 is > 35 mm. The R wave in aVL is 17 mm (1.7 mV). The ST and T waves are opposite in direction to the main deflection of the QRS complexes.

Right Ventricular Hypertrophy

Right ventricular hypertrophy (RVH) should be considered when the R/S ratio (height of the R wave divided by the height of the S wave) is > 1 in lead V1 in the absence of other causes or if the R wave in lead V1 is greater than 7 mm. When the right ventricular wall is quite thick and the pressure is high, there may be ST segment depression and asymmetric T wave inversions in leads V1 to V3 which is referred to as a strain pattern. Other causes of an R/S ratio > 1 in lead V1 may include posterior wall myocardial infarction, right bundle branch block and Wolf Parkinson White syndrome.

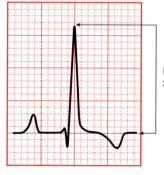

R wave is > 7 mm   OR   R/S ratio > 1

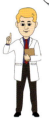

The ECG is insensitive for right and left ventricular hypertrophy.

Intraventricular Conduction Disturbances

Diseases involving the His-Purkinje system can give rise to changes in the morphology of the QRS complex and/or the frontal plane axis. The ECG pattern depends on what lesions are present within the His-Purkinje system.

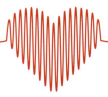

Right Bundle Branch Block

Right bundle branch block (RBBB) is the absence of conduction through the right bundle resulting in delayed activation of the right ventricle.

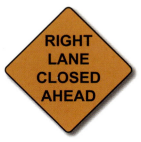

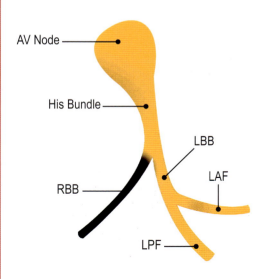

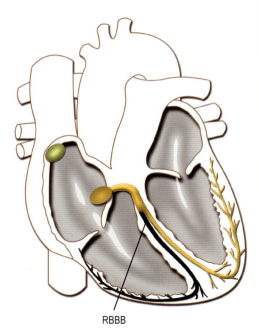

RBB - right bundle branch
LBB - left bundle branch
LAF - left anterior fascicle
LPF - left posterior fascicle
RBBB - right bundle branch block

conducted
non-conducted

Sequence of Ventricular Depolarization in Right Bundle Branch Block

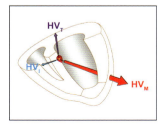

Normal

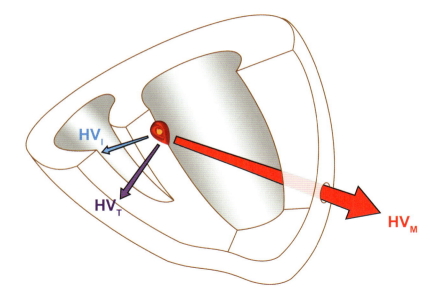

With RBBB, depolarization of the heart begins in the septum from left to right then spreads to the left ventricle and finally across to the right ventricle.

HV_I - Heart Vector Initial
HV_M - Heart Vector Main
HV_T - Heart Vector Terminal

The characteristic ECG patterns of right bundle branch block (RBBB) include:

1 Wide QRS complex ≥ 0.12 sec (3 small boxes).

2 The first part of the QRS complex will appear normal (septal q waves in the lateral leads) because the septum normally activates from left to right.

3 The late portion of the QRS complex is abnormal. A secondary R wave (R' or r') is commonly present resulting in a triphasic pattern or "bunny ears". This typical "bunny ears" pattern may not always be present. Instead, you may only see a dominant R wave in V1. One should remember that a tall and wide R wave in lead V1 in sinus rhythm is right bundle branch block with very few exceptions.

Lead V1

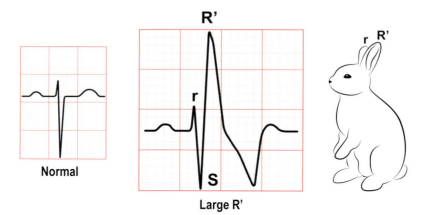

Wide, low amplitude terminal S wave in the anterolateral leads (I, aVL, V5 and V6). These shallow S waves represent delayed right ventricular conduction.

Lead V6

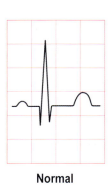

Normal

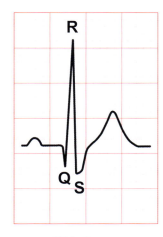

Wide S wave

 ST depression and T wave inversion in V1 (and possibly V2 and V3) due to abnormal repolarization. Also, the ST segments and T waves are opposite in direction to the main deflection of the QRS complex in these leads.

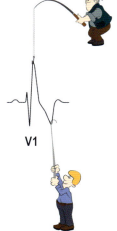

V1

The initial part of the QRS complex is not affected by complete right bundle branch block because it is a late conduction disorder.

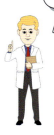

89

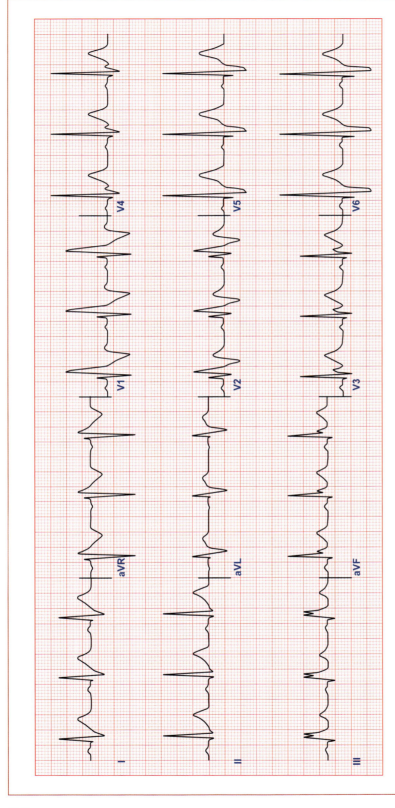

Sinus rhythm with right bundle branch block. The mean frontal plane QRS axis is normal. QRS duration of 0.16 sec. Lead V1 shows the typical rSR' pattern (rabbit ear sign). A wide terminal S wave is present in the lateral leads (I, aVL, V5 & V6). The right precordial leads (V1 and V2) show the ST and T waves opposite in direction to the main deflection of the QRS complexes.

Left Bundle Branch Block

Left bundle branch block (LBBB) is the absence of conduction through the left bundle resulting in delayed activation of the left ventricle.

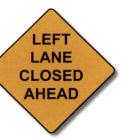

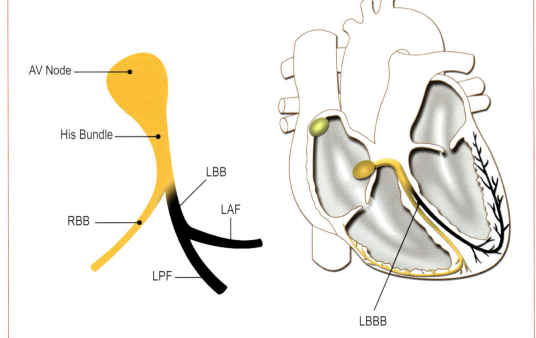

RBB - right bundle branch
LBB - left bundle branch
LAF - left anterior fascicle
LPF - left posterior fascicle
LBBB - left bundle branch block

▬▬▬ conducted
▬▬▬ non-conducted

Sequence of Ventricular Depolarization in Left Bundle Branch Block

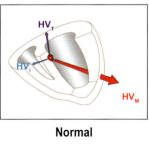

Normal

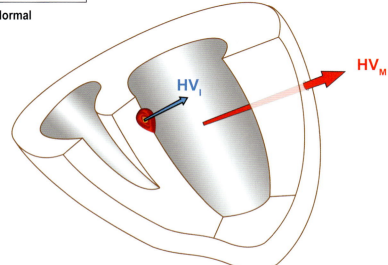

With LBBB, depolarization of the heart begins in the septum from right to left then spreads to the right ventricle and then across to the left ventricle. The terminal heart vector (HVt) is not shown here because it is also directed toward the left ventricle.

In the presence of LBBB, depolarization of the right ventricle has nearly no influence on the QRS complex.

HV_I - Heart Vector Initial
HV_M - Heart Vector Main
HV_T - Heart Vector Terminal

The characteristic ECG patterns of left bundle branch block (LBBB) include:

 Wide QRS complex ≥ 0.12 sec (3 small boxes).

 The lateral leads (I, aVL, V5 and V6) may show a tall R wave which is broad or notched ('M' shaped). Such tall R waves are not uniformly seen.

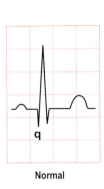

Normal

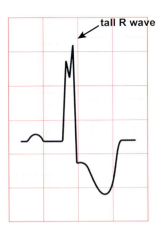

tall R wave

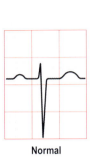 Usually, there are deep S waves in leads V1 to V3. The S wave may or may not be preceded by a small R wave. The genesis of the initial R wave, if present, is unclear. An S wave not preceded by an R wave is referred to as a QS complex.

Lead V1

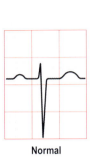

Normal

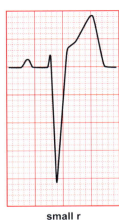

small r

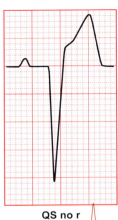

QS no r

The normal septal q waves typically seen in the lateral leads are absent. This is because the initial heart vector (HVi) is directed from right to left instead of the normal left to right to left during depolarization of the septum.

 Poor R wave progression in the precordial leads is common.

 The ST segments and T waves in the anterolateral leads (I, aVL, V5 and 6) are opposite in direction to the main deflection of the QRS complex due to abnormal repolarization.

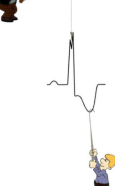

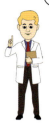

No septal q waves are present in leads V5 and V6 in complete LBBB.

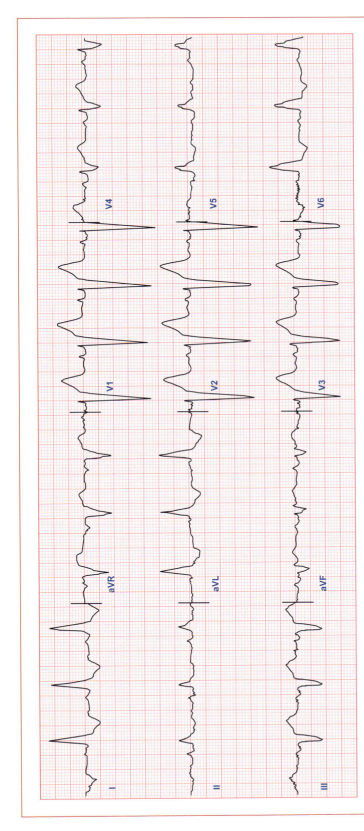

Sinus rhythm with complete left bundle branch block. The mean frontal plane QRS axis is normal. The QRS complex is wide and measures 0.12 sec. There are deep S waves in leads V1 to V3. The QRS complexes in leads V5 and V6 do not show septal q waves.

Right vs Left Bundle Branch Block

A simple rule to follow to distinguish RBBB from LBBB in the presence of a normally conducted sinus beat (not a premature beat) is to look at lead V1. If the main direction of the wide QRS complex is up then it is RBBB and if is down it is LBBB.

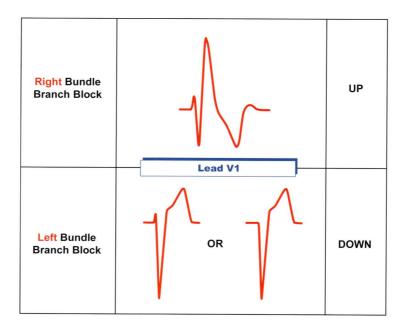

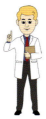

In a conducted beat with a wide QRS complex, a dominant R wave in lead V1 should be first considered as possible complete RBBB and a negative one complete LBBB. One should also look for other manifestations of intraventricular conduction disturbance.

Left Anterior Fascicular Block

Left anterior fascicular block (LAFB) is the absence of conduction through the left anterior fascicle of the left bundle branch resulting in activation of the left ventricle via the left posterior fascicle.

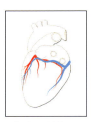

Lateral View

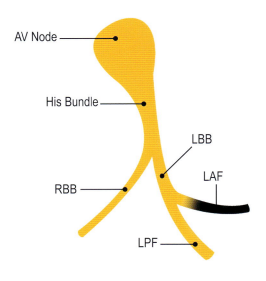

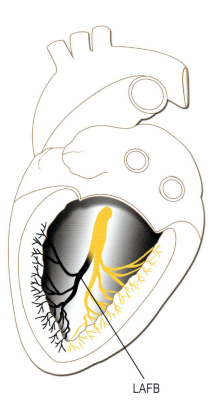

RBB - right bundle branch
LBB - left bundle branch
LAF - left anterior fascicle
LPF - left posterior fascicle
LAFB - left anterior fascicular block

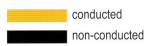

Sequence of Ventricular Depolarization in Left Anterior Fascicular Block

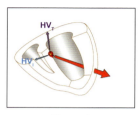

Normal

HV_I - Heart Vector Initial
HV_M - Heart Vector Main
HV_T - Heart Vector Terminal

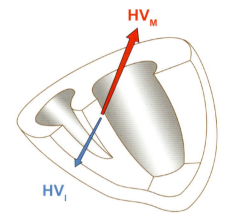

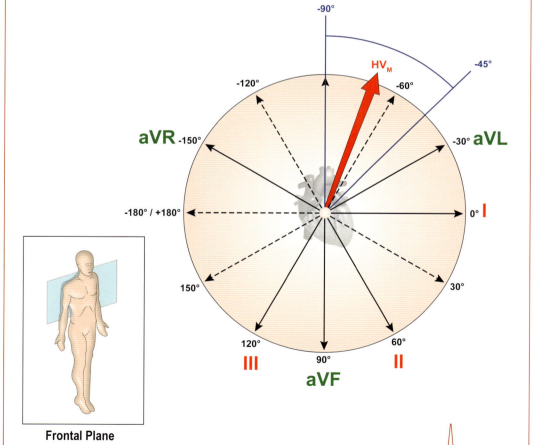

Frontal Plane

The characteristic patterns of left anterior fascicular block (also referred to as left anterior hemiblock) include:

1 There is left axis deviation (usually between -45° and -90°).

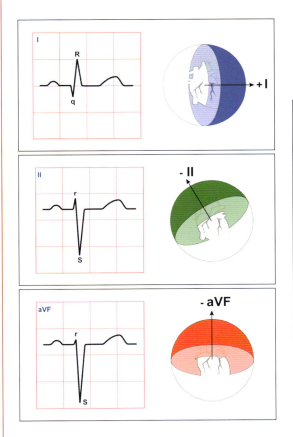
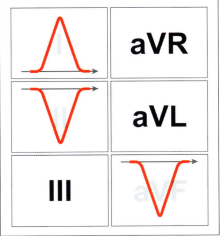

2 The QRS duration is < 0.12 sec.

A QRS that is positive in lead I, negative in lead aVF and equiphasic in lead II indicates an axis of -30° and immediately rules out LAFB.

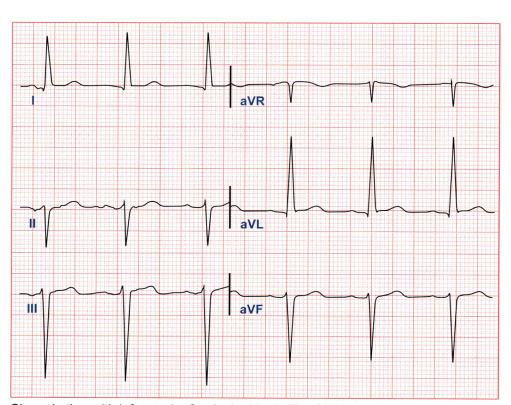

Sinus rhythm with left anterior fascicular block. The QRS duration is 0.10 sec. Lead I is upright, lead aVF is negative and lead II is predominantly negative indicating an axis more negative than -45 degrees.

Left Posterior Fascicular Block

Left posterior fascicular block (LPFB) is the absence of conduction through the left posterior fascicle of the left bundle branch resulting in activation of the left ventricle via the left anterior fascicle.

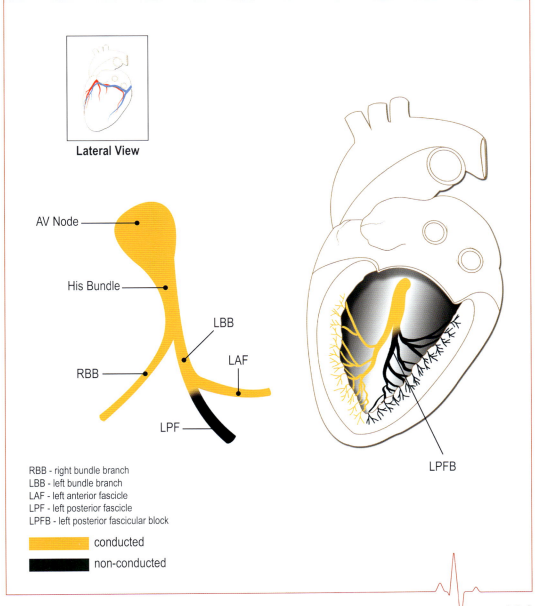

Lateral View

RBB - right bundle branch
LBB - left bundle branch
LAF - left anterior fascicle
LPF - left posterior fascicle
LPFB - left posterior fascicular block

conducted
non-conducted

Sequence of Ventricular Depolarization in Left Posterior Fascicular Block

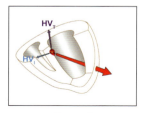

Normal

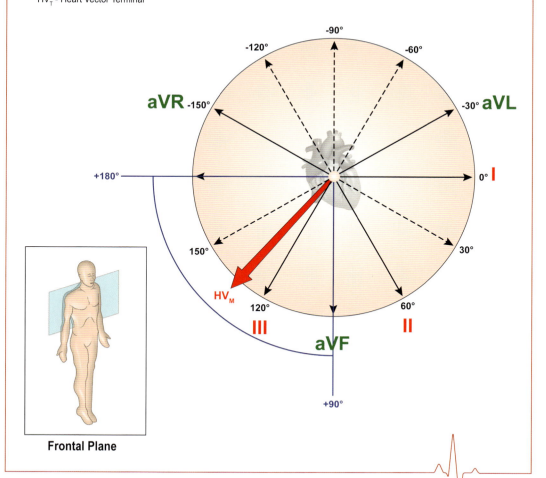

HV_I - Heart Vector Initial
HV_M - Heart Vector Main
HV_T - Heart Vector Terminal

Frontal Plane

102

The characteristic patterns of left posterior fascicular block (also referred to as left posterior hemiblock) include:

 There is right axis deviation (usually between +90° and +180°).

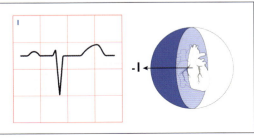

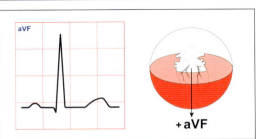

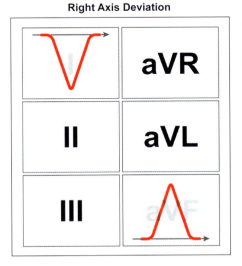

 The QRS duration is < 0.12 sec.

> This pattern is much less common than left anterior fascicular block. There are other causes of right axis deviation, including right ventricular hypertrophy and lateral wall myocardial infarction, and these must be excluded before a diagnosis of left posterior fascicular block can be made.

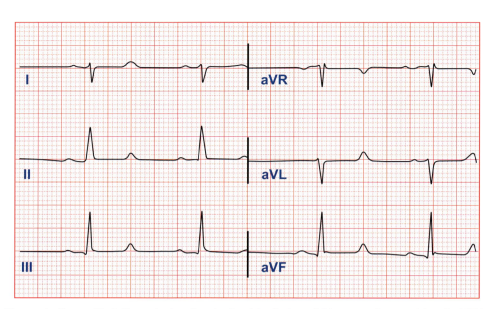

Sinus rhythm with left posterior fascicular block. Lead I is negative and lead aVF is positive indicating right axis deviation.

Bifascicular Block

Bifascicular block refers to an abnormality involving two parts of a three-pronged conduction system. There are three types of bifascicular block.

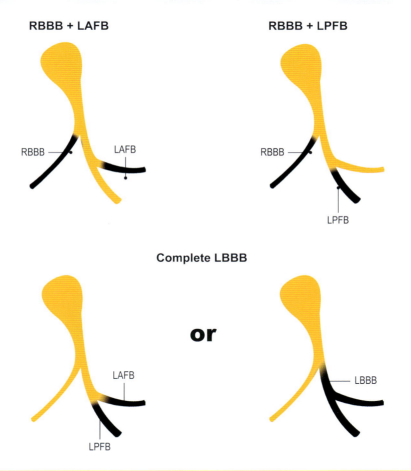

In order to diagnose bifascicular block involving the right bundle branch and one of the two left fascicles, the frontal plane axis must be examined.

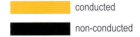

conducted
non-conducted

The characteristic ECG patterns of bifascicular block involving the right bundle and the left anterior fascicle include:

1 Right bundle branch block pattern.

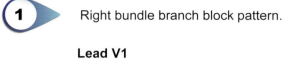

2 Left axis deviation (axis of -45° to -90°).

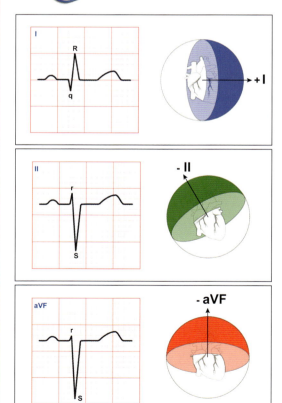

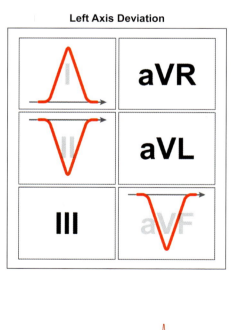

Left Axis Deviation

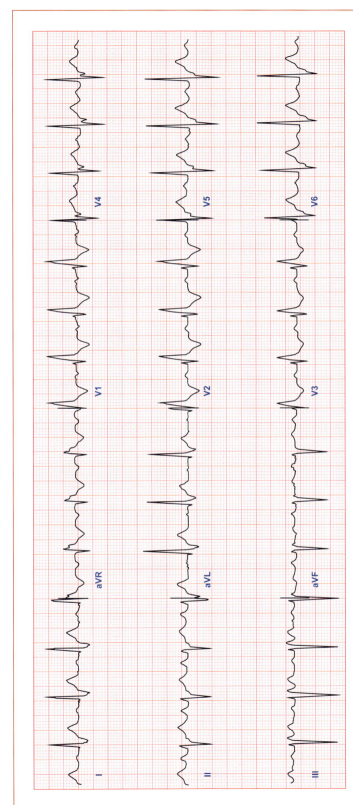

Sinus rhythm with a right bundle branch block. The mean frontal plane QRS axis is −45 degrees or more negative (lead I is up, lead aVF is down and the QRS is predominantly negative in lead II) which meets the diagnostic criteria for left anterior fascicular block. RBBB and LAFB constitutes bifascicular block.

Bifascicular block involving both the right bundle and left posterior fascicle is far less common and will not be shown here. In contrast, the frontal plane axis carries no diagnostic value in complete left bundle branch block.

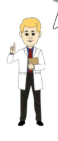

Bifascicular block implies ventricular activation by only one of three fascicles. Therefore, one should suspect intermittent malfunction of the third fascicle in a patient with dizzy spells or blackouts when the ECG suggests bifascicular block.

Myocardial Ischemia and Infarction

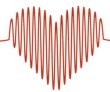

Myocardial Ischemia

Myocardial ischemia is a reduction in oxygenation of cardiac muscle due to inadequate coronary blood flow and may lead to a range of clinical presentations depending on its severity and duration.

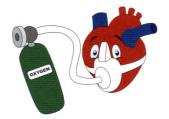

Myocardial ischemia of prolonged duration due to complete absence of blood flow will result in tissue injury and death. This is referred to as a myocardial infarction or "heart attack".

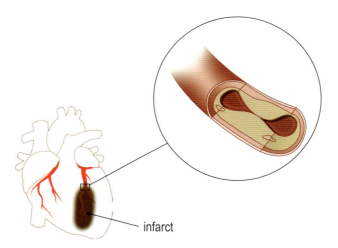

infarct

Myocardial infarctions can be classified into two types based on electrocardiographic presentation:

- **ST Elevation Myocardial Infarction (STEMI)**
- **Non ST Elevation Myocardial Infarction (NSTEMI)**

An ST elevation myocardial infarction is a life threatening emergency and often the result of complete occlusion of a coronary artery that requires rapid diagnosis.

Myocardial ischemia that is transient and does not result in tissue death is often, but not always, associated with symptoms.

Angina, short for angina pectoris, is a term often used to describe discomfort in the chest, jaw, shoulder, or arms attributable to myocardial ischemia.

Stable angina is a clinical syndrome characterized by angina or associated symptoms precipitated by certain activities and relieved by nitroglycerin. **Unstable angina** is characterized by symptoms that change or worsen and often occur at rest. Transient myocardial ischemia in the absence of symptoms is referred to as **silent ischemia**.

Unstable angina, ST elevation myocardial infarction and non ST elevation myocardial infarction are collectively referred to as **acute coronary syndromes**.

> Acute coronary syndromes can produce electrocardiographic abnormalities involving the ST segment and/or T wave. The appearance of the ECG depends on a number of factors including the anatomical location of ischemia, extent of myocardial involvement and the length of time the blood supply has been compromised.

ST Elevation Myocardial Infarction

The ECG "criteria" for a STEMI requires ST elevation (of at least 1 mm in the frontal leads and at least 2 mm in the precordial leads) in 2 anatomically contiguous leads.

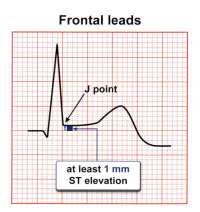

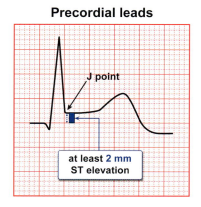

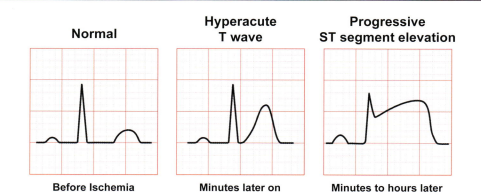

During the initial stages of a STEMI, hyper acute or "peaked" T waves may occur but this is very transient. The ST segment may initially appear concave but as it becomes more pronounced it becomes convex.

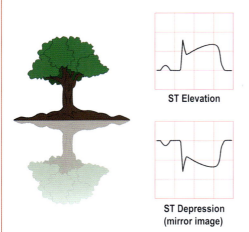

ST Elevation

ST Depression (mirror image)

ST elevation in one myocardial territory is often accompanied by ST depression in other myocardial territories. These ST depressions are referred to as reciprocal (mirror image) changes.

The anatomical location of the STEMI is determined by where on the 12-lead ECG the ST elevations are present:

ST Elevation in leads I, aVL, V5 and V6
(with reciprocal changes in II, III and aVF)

Lateral Wall STEMI

ST Elevation in leads V1 and V2

Septal Wall STEMI

ST Elevation in leads V3 and V4

Anterior Wall STEMI

ST Elevation in leads II, III and aVF
(with reciprocal changes in leads I and aVL and possibly the precordial leads)

Inferior Wall STEMI

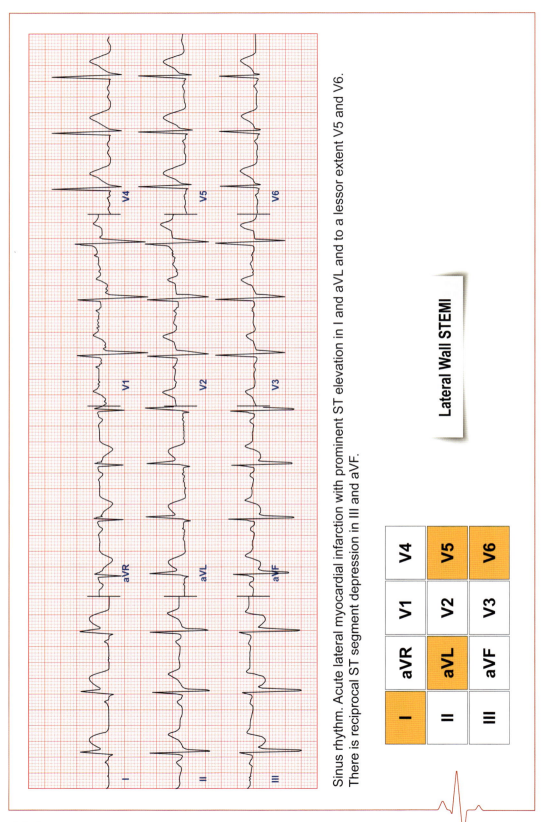

Sinus rhythm. Acute lateral myocardial infarction with prominent ST elevation in I and aVL and to a lessor extent V5 and V6. There is reciprocal ST segment depression in III and aVF.

Lateral Wall STEMI

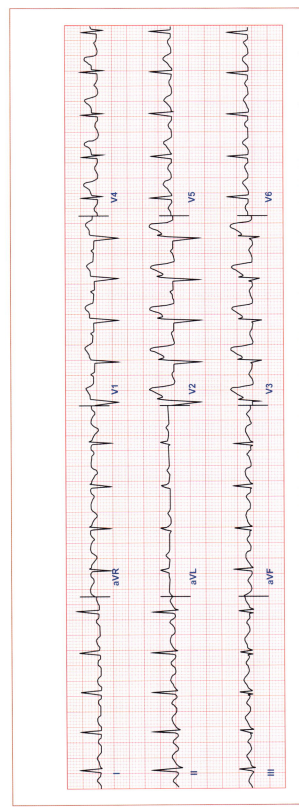

Sinus tachycardia. Acute anteroseptal myocardial infarction with prominent ST elevation in V1 though V4. There are Q waves in V1 and V2.

Anteroseptal Wall STEMI

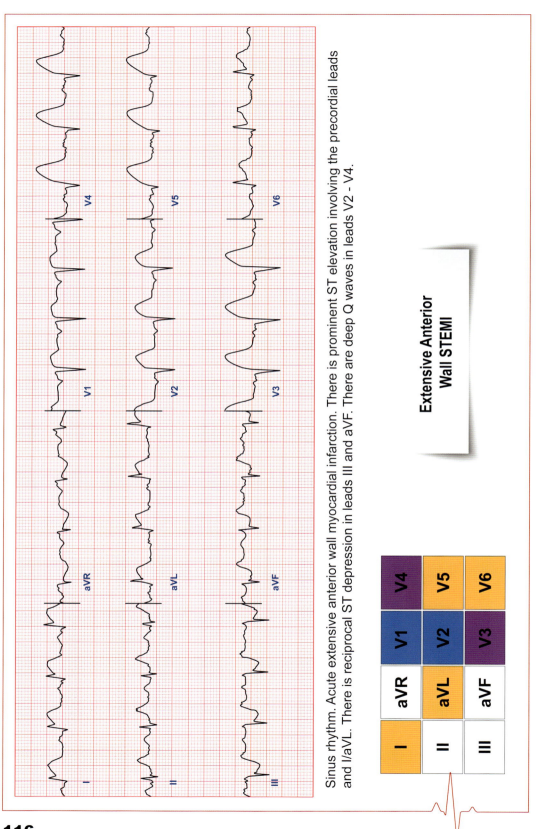

Sinus rhythm. Acute extensive anterior wall myocardial infarction. There is prominent ST elevation involving the precordial leads and I/aVL. There is reciprocal ST depression in leads III and aVF. There are deep Q waves in leads V2 - V4.

Extensive Anterior Wall STEMI

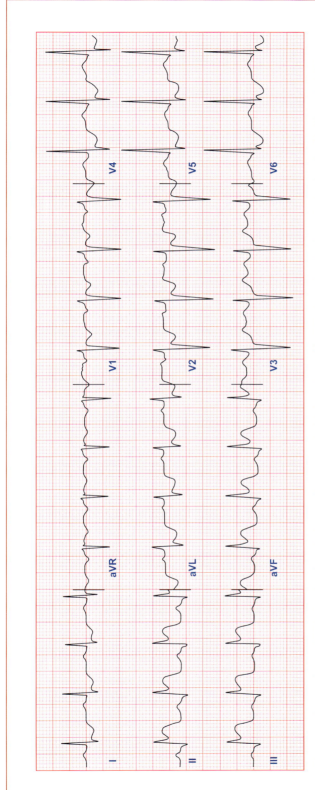

Sinus tachycardia at 100/min. Acute inferior wall myocardial infarction with ST elevation in the inferior leads (II, III and aVF). There is reciprocal ST depression in the anterior and lateral leads (I, aVL, V2 though V6).

Inferior Wall STEMI

A **Posterior Wall STEMI** may show on the ECG as a tall R wave in lead V1 and possibly lead V2, or an R/S ratio of > 1 in lead V1.

(Note: these particular ECG findings have also been observed with other conditions such as right ventricular hypertrophy and right bundle branch block)

A **Right Ventricular STEMI** may accompany inferior and posterior wall STEMI's. Right sided precordial leads are necessary when evaluating for a right ventricular STEMI. The best predictor of a right ventricular STEMI on ECG is ST elevation of 1 mm (1 small box) or more in lead V4R. This finding is often transient and may only be present for up to 12 hours after onset of symptoms.

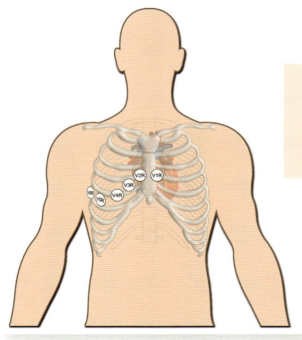

Right sided precordial leads (V1R to V6R) are positioned in a mirror image fashion to the standard left sided precordial leads.

In a suspected STEMI, serial ECG's are essential to determine the evolution of the acute ischemic event.

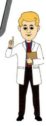

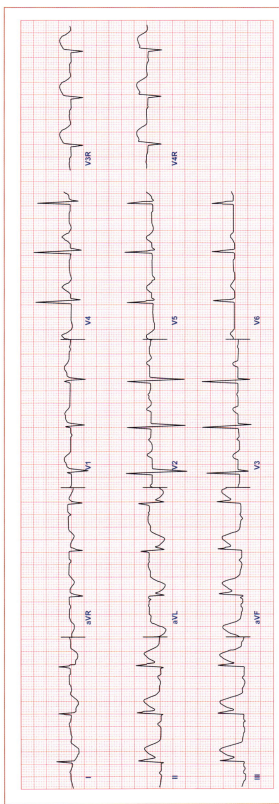

Sinus rhythm. Acute inferior wall myocardial infarction with prominent ST elevation in II, III and aVF. There is also slight ST elevation in lead V1 suggesting a right ventricular infarction. Leads V3R and V4R show > 1 mm ST elevation confirming an acute right ventricular myocardial infarction. Also note the reciprocal changes in leads I and aVL.

Non-ST Elevation Myocardial Infarction and Unstable Angina

Unstable angina (UA) and **non ST elevation myocardial infarction** (NSTEMI) are often difficult to tell apart at initial evaluation. Both can produce the same spectrum of ECG changes ranging from no abnormalities to ST segment depression and/or T wave inversions. These ST/T wave abnormalities are often referred to as "ST-T wave changes". What distinguishes the two in the end is the presence or absence of an elevated cardiac biomarker (elevation in cardiac biomarkers may not be detectable for up to 12 hours after presenting symptoms). Biomarkers are elevated with a NSTEMI and not elevated with unstable angina.

Possible ECG findings associated with NSTEMI and unstable angina include:

ST segment depression that is either downsloping or horizontal (the normal ST segment starts at the isoelectric line and curves smoothly upwards into the T wave). The extent and magnitude of the ST segment depression correlates with the severity of ischemia.

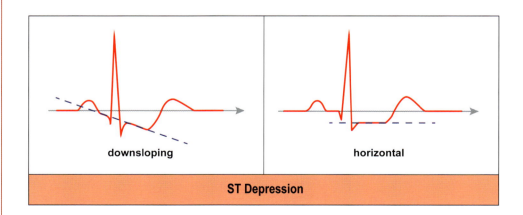

Abnormalities involving the T wave including T wave inversion and T wave flattening. The T wave inversions are symmetrical in shape (downsloping limb is a mirror image of the upsloping limb).

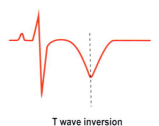

T wave inversion   T wave flattening

3 An important subgroup of patients with severe disease can present with either deeply inverted symmetrical T waves (often diffuse) or biphasic T waves (positive initial deflection) in leads V1 to V3.

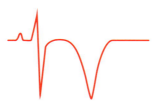 or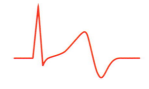

Deep T wave inversion   Biphasic T waves

> The ST segment and T wave can appear normal in the setting of UA and a NSTEMI.

121

ST elevation or abnormal Q waves are not seen with NSTEMI's or unstable angina. Having an old ECG for comparison can be very valuable to determine if these ECG findings are new or longstanding.

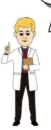

Additional ECG recordings can be valuable with any changes in symptoms especially when the initial ECG is normal or the changes are subtle.

Other Causes of Non-ischemic T wave Inversions*

- Left bundle branch block
- Right bundle branch block
- Left ventricular hypertrophy
- Right ventricular hypertrophy
- Paced rhythm
- Pulmonary disease
- Cardiomyopathy
- Wolf Parkinson White syndrome

* Not a comprehensive list

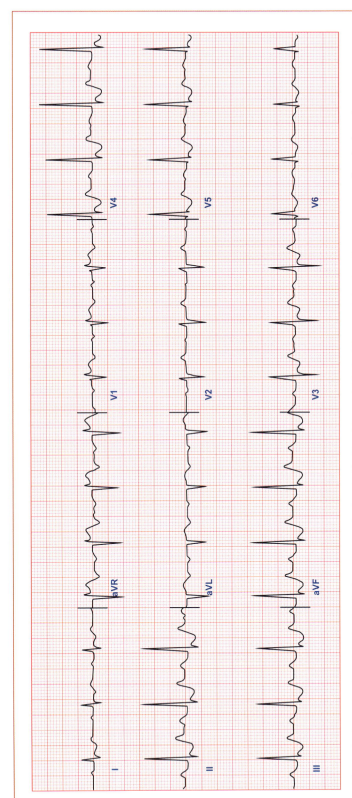

Normal sinus rhythm. Marked ST depression in leads II, III, aVF and V3 to V5 consistent with severe cardiac ischemia.

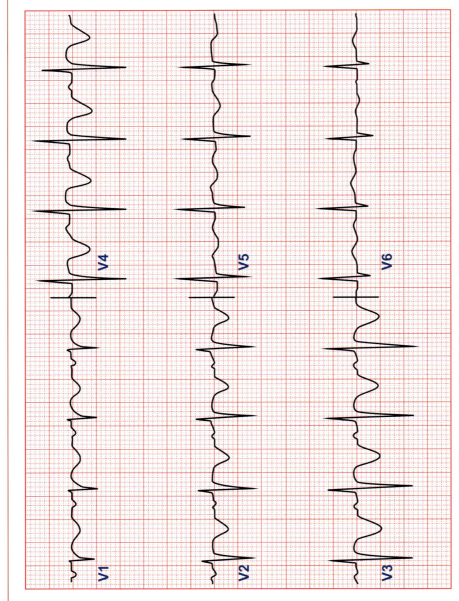

Sinus rhythm. Deep T wave inversions in leads V2 to V4 highly suggestive of severe myocardial ischemia.

Pathological Q Waves

A common consequence of a STEMI on the ECG is the formation of "pathological" Q waves. They are the result of an absence of electrical activity in the area of the heart that was damaged.

Q or QS waves may appear as early as 1-2 hours after onset of a STEMI or may take greater than 24 hours.

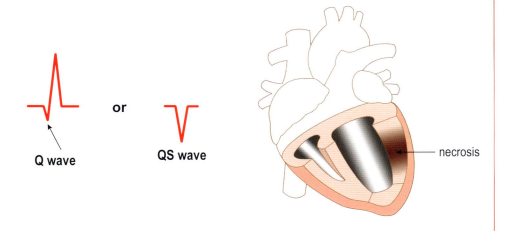

The electrocardiographic changes associated with a prior myocardial infarction include:

  Any Q wave or QS complex in leads V2 and V3 that measures ≥ 0.02 sec.

  Any Q wave or QS complex in two leads of a continuous lead grouping (I and aVL; II, III and aVF; V1 to V6) with a duration of > 0.03 sec and > 0.1 mV deep.

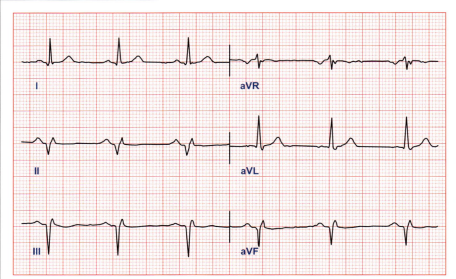

Sinus rhythm with prominent Q waves in II, III and aVF consistent with an old inferior wall MI. There is also T wave flattening in the same leads.

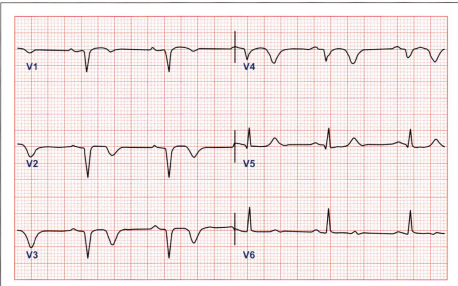

Sinus rhythm with prominent Q waves in V1 to V4 consistent with an old anteroseptal wall MI. There is prominent T wave inversion in V2 to V4.

It is important to remember that not all Q waves are a consequence of a myocardial infarction!

Normal Q Waves

- Small septal q waves are commonly seen in leads I, aVL, V5 and V6 as a result of normal septal depolarization.

- Small q waves may also be seen in leads III and aVF and are less than 1/3rd the amplitude of the R wave.

Myocardial Infarction and Bundle Branch Block

Identifying a **STEMI in the presence of a bundle branch block** is difficult because of the abnormal ST segments and T waves. The currently used algorithms to identify a STEMI in this setting of a bundle branch block fall short.

Identifying a **prior myocardial infarction in the presence of a bundle branch block** depends on the location of the block. As a rule, an old myocardial infarction cannot usually be diagnosed if a left bundle branch block is present because a left bundle branch block affects the initial part of the QRS complex. In contrast, an old myocardial infarction can be seen if a right bundle branch block is present because the initial part of the QRS complex is not affected by the right bundle branch block.

Other Causes of ST Elevation

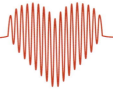

Early Repolarization

Early repolarization is characterized by J point elevation (J point is the junction between the end of the QRS complex and the beginning of the ST segment), ST elevation with upper concavity and prominent T waves in two contiguous leads.

J point elevation can manifest as either end-QRS slurring or notching. Historically, early repolarization has been thought to be a benign entity, however, more recent reports suggest rare forms may be associated with ventricular arrhythmias.

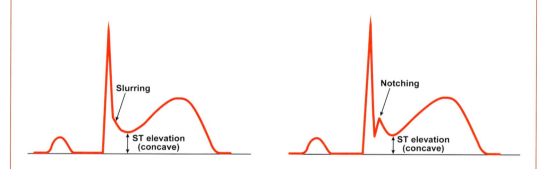

Some features that may help distinguish early repolarization from a STEMI include:

1 The ST segments are typically concave upwards.

2 There is absence of reciprocal ST depression.

3 The ST elevations remain fairly constant (in contrast to ischemia that usually produces an evolving pattern).

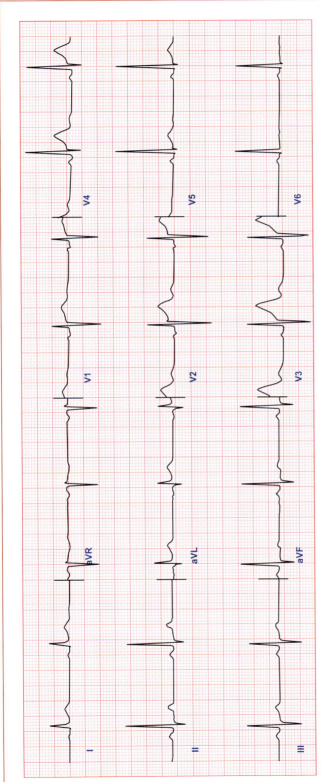

Sinus bradycardia with early repolarization. Note the concave ST segments in leads aVL and V2 - V4. This must not be confused with disease with pathological ST elevation.

Pericarditis

Pericarditis refers to inflammation of the pericardium, the fibroelastic sac surrounding the heart. The outer layer of the heart, referred to as the epicardium, is also the innermost layer of the pericardium and when inflamed can produce repolarization abnormalities including ST segment elevation.

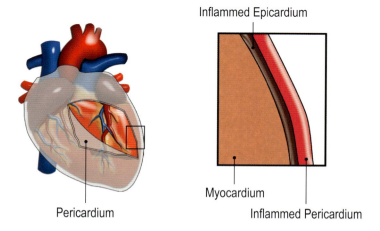

Useful electrocardiographic clues to differentiate pericarditis from a STEMI include:

1 The ST segment elevations usually involve most leads and do not correspond with any specific myocardial territory.

2 The ST segment elevations are typically concave upwards (saddle-shaped) as opposed to convex typically seen with a STEMI.

3 The ST segment elevations are usually < 5 mm.

4 There are no associated reciprocal changes.

> ST elevation in leads I and II essentially rules out myocardial ischemia.

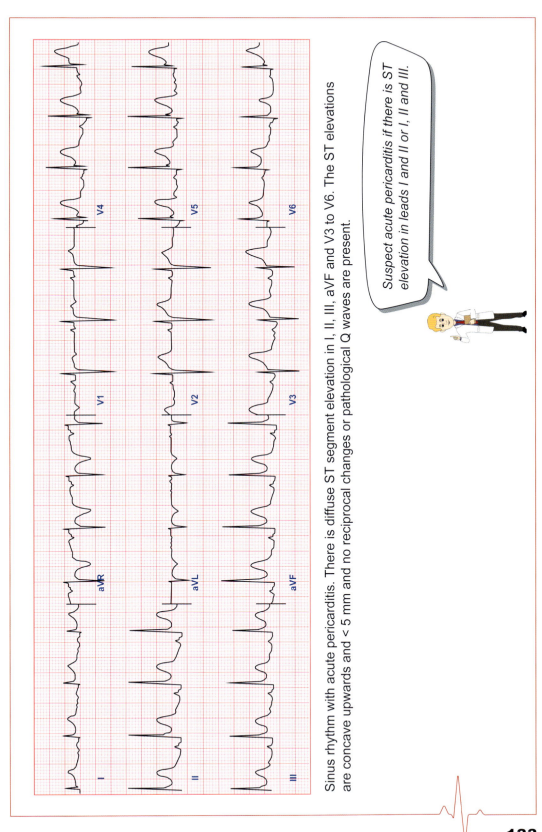

Sinus rhythm with acute pericarditis. There is diffuse ST segment elevation in I, II, III, aVF and V3 to V6. The ST elevations are concave upwards and < 5 mm and no reciprocal changes or pathological Q waves are present.

Suspect acute pericarditis if there is ST elevation in leads I and II or I, II and III.

Left Ventricular Aneurysm

A left ventricular aneurysm is a localized area of thinned left ventricular wall that bulges or does not move during systole and is commonly the result of an extensive myocardial infarction. The ECG in the precordial leads shows persistent ST segment elevation, usually convex in form, and Q waves of old infarction.

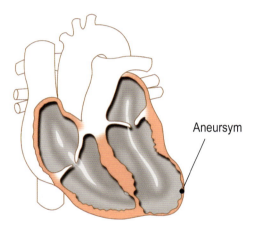

Aneursym

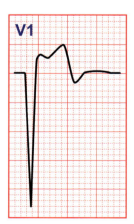
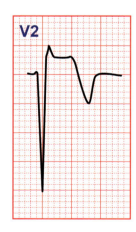
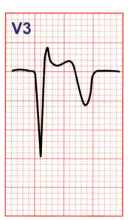

Brugada Syndrome

Brugada syndrome is a genetic condition characterized by "coved" type ST elevation of ≥ 2 mm (0.2 mV) in leads V1 and V2 and associated with malignant ventricular tachyarrhythmias and an increased risk for sudden cardiac death.

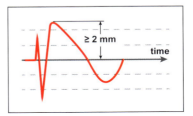

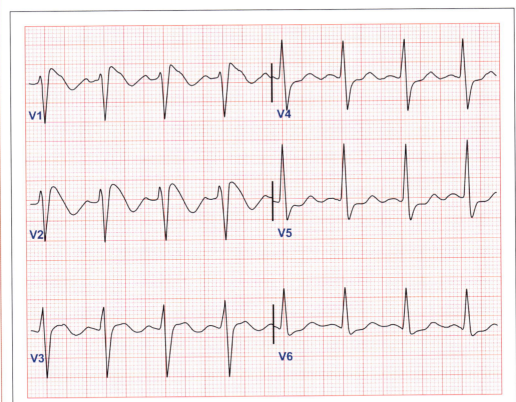

Sinus rhythm with prominent coved ST elevations > 2 mm in V1 and V2 diagnostic of Brugada syndrome.

Concave vs Convex Patterns of ST Elevation

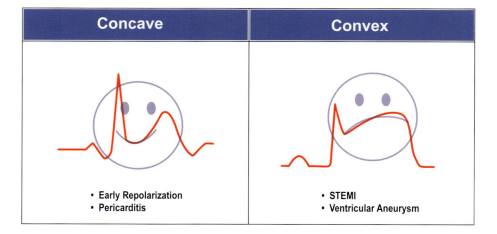

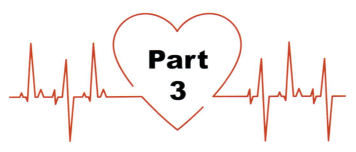

Part 3

Rhythm Disturbances

Classification of Arrhythmias

Over the years, arrhythmias have been classified in a number of ways -- site of origin, mechanism of action, bradyarrhythmias vs tachyarrhythmias, regular vs irregular rhythm, sustained vs unsustained, permanent vs paroxysmal to name a few. There is no single classification that can be applied uniformly to all rhythm disorders.

In this book, the rhythm disorders will be presented in the following order:

Atrial & Junctional Arrhythmias

Supraventricular Tachyarrhythmias

Wolf Parkinson White Syndrome

Ventricular Arrhythmias

Ventricular Tachyarrhythmias

Atrioventricular Conduction Blocks

Atrial and Junctional Arrhythmias

These refer to narrow QRS complex (QRS is not prolonged except in the presence of an intraventricular conduction disturbance) arrhythmias originating in the atria (SA node included) or AV junction (defined as low atria, AV node and His Bundle) with a HR < 100/min.

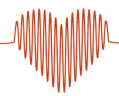

Sinus Bradycardia

Sinus bradycardia has all of the characteristics of normal sinus rhythm except that the rate is < 60/min.

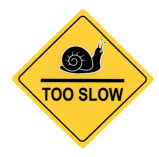

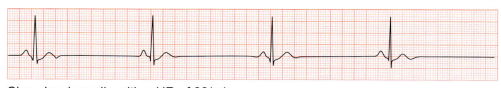

Sinus bradycardia with a HR of 30/min.

Sinus Arrhythmia

Sinus arrhythmia is a manifestation of normal sinus rhythm with some irregularity in the rate. There may be irregular variations in the PP intervals as much as or more than 0.12 sec. The PR intervals are usually constant with no change in the configuration of the P waves. There are 2 types -- respiratory and non-respiratory. The respiratory form is more common and discussed below.

Respiratory Form

The variation in rate is a normal physiological response and results from respiration which leads to changes in the autonomic nervous system. Inspiration results in a slight increase in heart rate and expiration results in a slight decrease in heart rate.

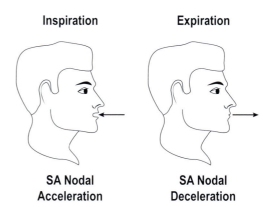

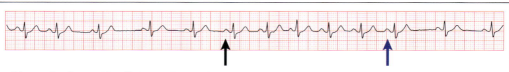

Sinus rhythm with slight variation in the rate indicating sinus arrhythmia. The heart rate begins to speed up (black arrow) during inspiration and slows down (blue arrow) during expiration.

141

Sinoatrial Exit Block

With sinoatrial exit block, the pacemaker cells within the sinoatrial (SA) node function normally according to their intrinsic timing and are able to generate an impulse on time. However, the impulse cannot be conducted through the transitional cells within the node and into the surrounding atrial tissue. There are several forms of sinoatrial exit block, however, the only visible form on ECG is second degree (partial) exit block.

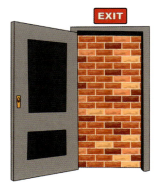

The characteristic ECG patterns of second degree sinoatrial exit block:

1 Absence of a P wave at the expected time of the sinus cycle resulting in a pause.

2 The PP duration of the pause is an exact multiple of the preceding normal PP interval.

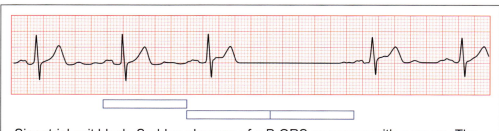

Sinoatrial exit block. Sudden absence of a P-QRS sequence with a pause. The PP interval encompassing the pause is exactly twice the previous PP interval (short bar).

Sinus Arrest

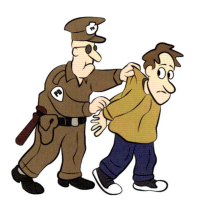

With sinus arrest, there is significant slowing of sinus discharge resulting in the absence of a sinus P wave and a pause which is not a multiple of the basic PP interval. The pause may or may not be followed by an escape rhythm. Escape rhythms that manifest in the setting of sinus slowing are most commonly from the AV junction.

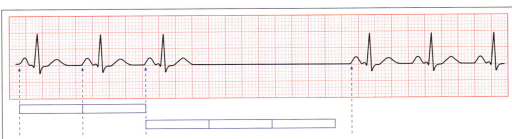

Sinus arrest. There is a pause and the long P-P interval is not an exact multiple of the previous shorter P-P intervals (short bar).

Atrial Premature Complexes

An atrial premature complex (APC) occurs when there is premature activation of the atria from an impulse originating from an atrial ectopic focus and not the sinoatrial node. The appearance on the ECG depends on the timing and location of the ectopic focus. The atrial premature impulse can be conducted normally to the ventricles, aberrantly (with an intra-ventricular conduction delay) or not conducted at all through the AV junction to the ventricle.

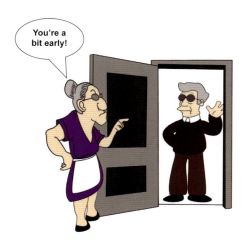

The characteristic ECG patterns of a normally conducted atrial premature impulse:

1 The P wave starts earlier in the cycle.

2 The P wave shows a different configuration compared to the normal sinus P wave.

3 Usually, a premature atrial impulse conducts retrogradely and resets the SA node. As a result, the PP interval encompassing the APC (from the P wave before the APC to the P wave after the APC) measures less than twice the PP interval between two normally conducted sinus beats. This ECG pattern is referred to as an "APC with a non-compensatory pause."

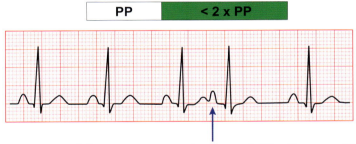

Sinus rhythm with an atrial premature complex (arrow). The P wave of the APC has a different configuration from the sinus P waves and is followed by a normal appearing QRS complex. The PP interval encompassing the APC (green bar) is less than double the prevailing sinus PP interval (white bar) and is due to resetting of the sinus node.

A premature or early atrial impulse may <u>not</u> conduct to the ventricles if the AV node is in a refractory state (not able to conduct).

The characteristic ECG patterns of a <u>non-conducted</u> atrial premature impulse (often referred to as a "blocked" atrial premature complex):

 The P wave, if visible, is not followed by a QRS complex.

 The P wave may be buried within the T wave and invisible or superimposed on the T wave causing the T wave to appear "peaked" or have a "camel hump" appearance.

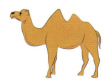

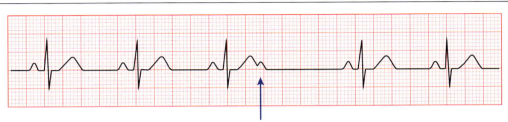

Sinus rhythm with a non-conducted atrial premature complex (arrow). The P wave is superimposed on the T wave. This does not reflect disease but the pause may be misinterpreted for other conditions. Mysterious pauses may occur when the P wave is not visible because it is buried in the T wave.

One should remember that the commonest cause of a pause on the ECG is a "blocked" atrial premature impulse.

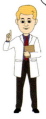

A non-conducted atrial premature impulse is a physiological phenomenon.

A premature or early atrial impulse may reach the ventricular conduction system when part of it is still in its refractory state.

The characteristic ECG patterns of an <u>aberrantly conducted</u> atrial premature impulse :

 Same features as a conducted atrial premature complex except that the QRS complex has a bundle branch block pattern (RBBB more common than LBBB).

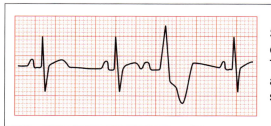

Sinus rhythm with an aberrantly conducted atrial premature complex. The wide QRS complex results from aberrancy when the His-Purkinje system is still in a refractory state.

Wandering Atrial Pacemaker

With wandering atrial pacemaker, the origin of the atrial impulse shifts or "wanders" between the sinoatrial node and at least three other ectopic foci located within the area and/or AV junction.

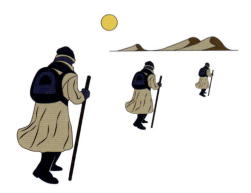

The characteristic ECG patterns of wandering atrial pacemaker:

1. There are at least three distinctly different P waves.

2. PR intervals can vary with shifting around of the atrial ectopic foci.

3. Irregular PP and RR intervals resulting in an irregular rhythm.

4. Heart rate < 100/min by definition.

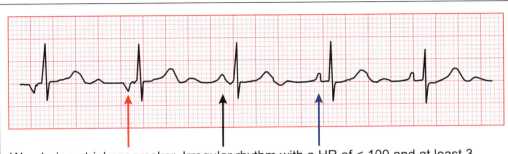

Wandering atrial pacemaker. Irregular rhythm with a HR of < 100 and at least 3 different P wave configurations (red, black and blue arrows).

147

Junctional Arrhythmias

These rhythms originate from the AV junction and include the following:

- Junctional Premature Complex
- Junctional Escape Rhythm
- Accelerated Junctional Rhythm
- Junctional Tachycardia

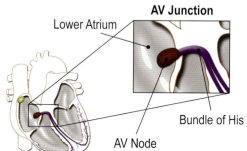

An impulse from the AV junction will activate the ventricles in a normal **anterograde** fashion resulting in a narrow QRS complex (unless there is aberrant conduction because of marked prematurity). In addition, an AV junctional impulse can sometimes activate the atria via **retrograde** conduction.

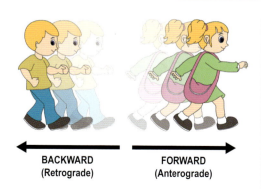

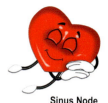

When retrograde conduction happens, the sinus node is suppressed so that no normal sinus-generated (anterograde) P waves are present.

Visibility of the retrograde P waves will depend on whether retrograde activation of the atria occurs before, during or after anterograde activation of the ventricles.

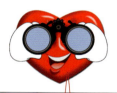

Retrograde P waves are inverted in leads II, III and aVF

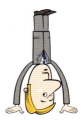

Possible locations of the P wave in a junctional arrhythmia:

"Hidden" in the QRS

The duration of anterograde and retrograde conduction is similar. There are no visible P waves.

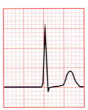

After the QRS

Retrograde atrial activation occurs after anterograde ventricular activation. The P waves are **inverted** in leads II, III and aVF.

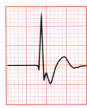

Before the QRS

Retrograde atrial activation occurs before anterograde ventricular activation. The P waves are **inverted** in leads II, III and aVF.

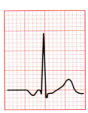

If retrograde conduction from the AV junction is blocked, the sinoatrial node is no longer suppressed and sinus rhythm will be maintained. As a result, atrial activation is normal and occurs independently of ventricular activation. The ECG is characterized by the presence of sinus P waves that bear no relation to the QRS complexes. The P waves can be described as "marching" though the QRS complexes. This situation is called **AV dissociation.**

Junctional Premature Complex

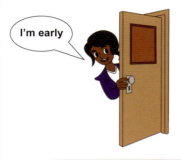

Junctional premature complexes occur when an impulse from the AV junction arises prematurely before the next expected sinus impulse. The relationship between the P and QRS complex is as described above in terms of a single junctional complex.

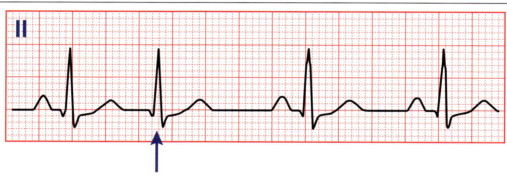

Sinus rhythm with a junctional premature complex (blue arrow). The QRS is narrow and is not associated with a visible P wave.

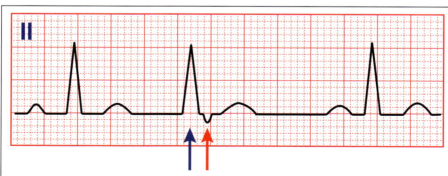

Sinus rhythm with a junctional premature complex (blue arrow) and an inverted retrograde P wave (red arrow) after the QRS complex.

150

Junctional Rhythms

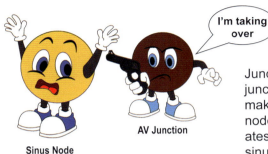

Junctional rhythms occur when the AV junction takes over as the primary pacemaker site either because the sinoatrial node has failed or the AV junction generates a rhythm that is faster than normal sinus rhythm.

Junctional rhythms are classified according to rate as follows:

- **Junctional Escape Rhythm:** 40-60/min. The AV junction becomes an escape pacemaker if the sinoatrial node fails to fire. It serves as a safety (passive) mechanism in contrast to faster functional rhythms (below) that actively take over control of the heart rate.
- **Accelerated Junctional Rhythm:** 60-100/min.
- **Junctional Tachycardia:** > 100/min.

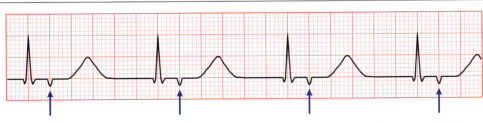

Junctional escape rhythm at a HR of 50/min with visible inverted retrograde P waves (arrows) after each QRS complex.

151

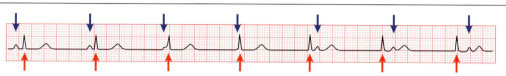

Junctional escape rhythm with AV dissociation. The sinus P waves (blue arrows) bear no relation to the QRS complexes (red arrows). The atrial rate is slightly slower than the ventricular rate.

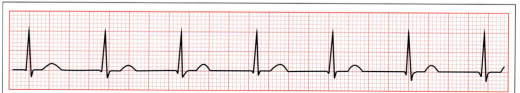

Accelerated junction rhythm. The heart rate is 80/min and there are no visible P waves.

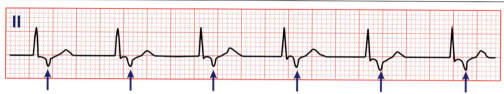

Accelerated junction rhythm. The heart rate is 88/min and there are retrograde P waves (arrows) after each QRS complex.

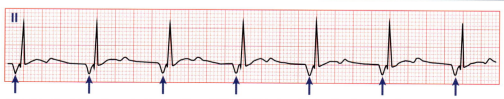

Accelerated junction rhythm with a HR of 75/min. Note the inverted retrograde P waves (arrows) before the QRS complexes.

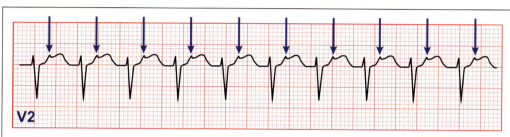

Junctional tachycardia with a heart rate of 136/min. Note the retrograde P waves (arrows) which are upright in lead V2 (usually inverted in leads II, III and aVF).

Supraventricular Tachyarrhythmias

These refer to narrow QRS complex arrhythmias originating in the atria or AV junction with a HR > 100/min.

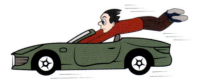
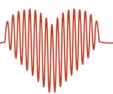

Sinus Tachycardia

Sinus tachycardia has all of the characteristics of normal sinus rhythm except that the rate is > 100/min. The PR interval shortens with tachycardia.

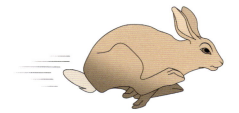

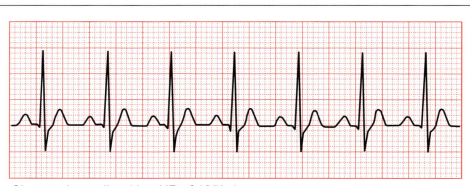

Sinus tachycardia with a HR of 125/min.

Focal Atrial Tachycardia

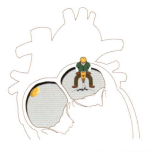

Focal atrial tachycardia is an ectopic atrial rhythm whose appearance on ECG depends on the ventricular rate and on AV conduction.

The characteristic ECG patterns of focal atrial tachycardia:

 The atrial rate can range from 100/min to as high as 250/min. The rate is commonly faster than 150/min.

 The ventricular rate is usually regular and may vary based on the behavior of the AV junction. When the atrial rates are very high and/or there is disease or medication affecting the AV node, intermittent AV block may be present resulting in more P waves than QRS complexes.

 P waves, when visible, appear different from normal sinus P waves. With very fast ventricular rates, the P waves are often not visible because they are "buried" in the QRS complex or T wave.

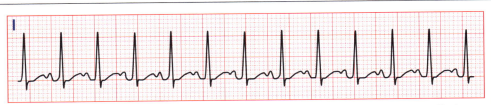

The tracing resembles sinus tachycardia with a HR of 165. The tachycardia is unlikely to originate from the sinus node because of the very fast rate. The very rapid rate and P wave preceding the QRS complex strongly suggests the presence of focal atrial tachycardia.

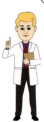

Focal atrial tachycardia can be mistaken for sinus tachycardia when the P wave precedes the QRS complex

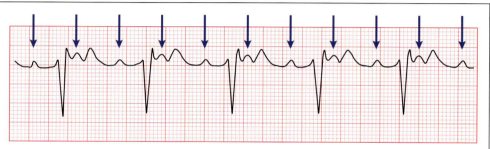

Atrial tachycardia with 2:1 AV block. The P waves (arrows) are clearly visible, the atrial rate is 135/min and every second P wave is conducted to the ventricle. The QRS is > 0.12 sec indicative of an intraventricular conduction disorder. This rhythm can be mistaken for sinus tachycardia with 2:1 AV block. The diagnosis was proven during an electrophysiology study.

Multifocal Atrial Tachycardia

Multifocal atrial tachycardia consists of multiple sites of competing ectopic atrial activity like wandering atrial pacemaker except that the rate is > 100/min.

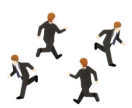

The characteristic ECG patterns of multifocal atrial tachycardia:

 There are at least three distinctly different P waves.

 PR intervals vary depending on the site of the ectopic foci.

 There is an "irregularly irregular" rhythm. An "irregularly irregular" rhythm refers to an irregular rhythm (inconsistent RR intervals) where there is no identifiable pattern within the irregularity. There is no predictability or pattern to the RR intervals. This is opposed to a "regularly irregular" rhythm where there is an identifiable pattern within the irregularity. The illustration below helps differentiate the two types of irregular rhythms. The different colored shapes represent different RR intervals.

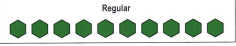
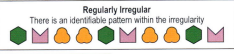
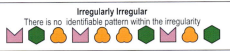

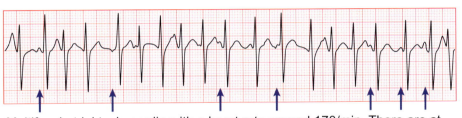

Multifocal atrial tachycardia with a heart rate around 170/min. There are at least 3 P waves (arrows) of varying configuration and the rhythm is irregular.

157

Atrial Fibrillation

With atrial fibrillation, there are numerous micro re-entrant circuits within the atria resulting in disorganized and chaotic electrical activation of the atria.

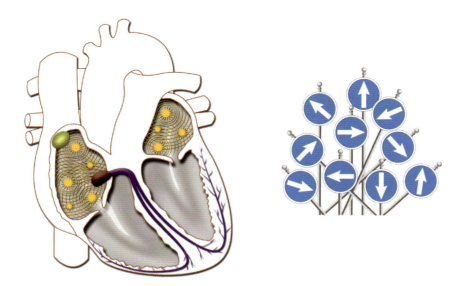

The characteristic ECG patterns of atrial fibrillation:

1 Instead of P waves, there are very small irregular "f" or fibrillatory waves which occur at a frequency of 350-600/min. This typically creates an undulating baseline in terms of amplitude and cycle length. The baseline undulation may be quite subtle (note - with longstanding atrial fibrillation, the f waves may be absent with a flat appearing baseline).

2 The QRS complexes are typically narrow unless there is an intraventricular conduction disturbance.

3 Irregularly irregular rhythm.

4 The ventricular rate can be slow, within normal range, or fast according to the status of AV conduction.

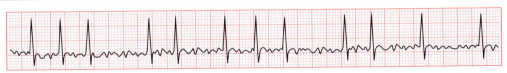

Atrial fibrillation with an irregular ventricular rate. The P waves are absent and replaced by low amplitude, high frequency f waves.

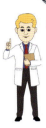

Atrial fibrillation is the commonest irregular rhythm without visible P waves. A rhythm strip must be examined to reveal constantly changing RR intervals.

The normal AV node cannot conduct all the fast atrial impulses transmitted to the AV junction. This physiological "brake" limits the transmitted ventricular rate of new onset atrial fibrillation usually to 140 - 160/min or occasionally as high as 200/min. This is often described as atrial fibrillation with rapid ventricular response.

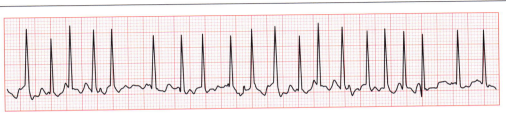

Atrial fibrillation with a rapid irregular ventricular response of 190/min.

When the ventricular response is very rapid, at first glance the rhythm may appear regular. However, on closer inspection, it will be found to be irregular. This irregularity is best ascertained with calipers.

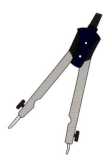

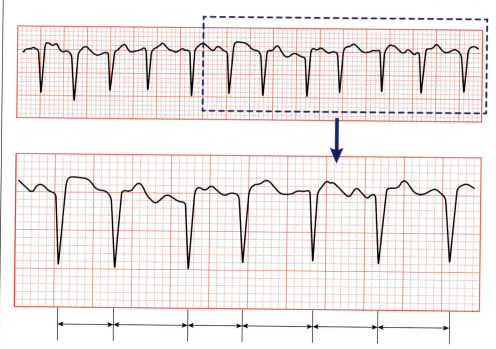

At first glance, the rhythm appears to be a regular tachycardia. However, closer inspection reveals that there is irregularity in the ventricular cycles consistent with atrial fibrillation with an irregular rapid ventricular response.

Atrial fibrillation is often seen with a normal or slow ventricular response. The most likely explanation is that the patient is being treated with medication designed to slow down AV nodal conduction.

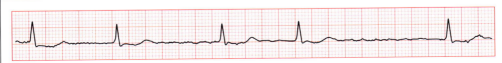

Atrial fibrillation with a slow irregular ventricular rate of about 50/min. The baseline appears flat without clear f waves. Delayed AV conduction from disease or medications will slow the ventricular rate.

Atrial Flutter

Atrial flutter is caused by a macro-reentrant loop phenomenon confined to the right atrium in most cases.

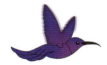

The characteristic ECG patterns of atrial flutter:

1 Instead of seeing P waves, you see "flutter" waves which occur at a frequency of 240 - 300/min, often around 300/min. These "flutter" waves closely resemble the blade of a handsaw.

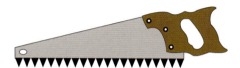

2 Atrial flutter is classified into typical and atypical (atypical forms are rare). There are 2 types of typical flutter -- anti-clockwise and clockwise. Anti-clockwise constitutes 90% of typical atrial flutter. With anticlockwise flutter, the isoelectric line is not visible and the flutter waves are inverted in leads II, III and aVF because activation moves from the inferior to the superior parts of the atrium.

Anti-Clockwise Atrial Flutter

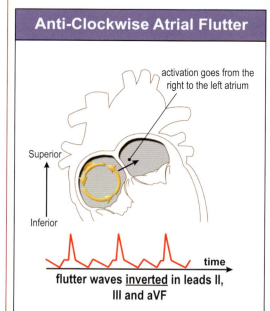

flutter waves <u>inverted</u> in leads II, III and aVF

Clockwise Atrial Flutter

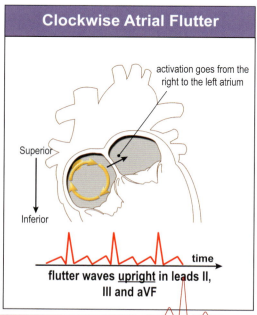

flutter waves <u>upright</u> in leads II, III and aVF

162

The ventricular rate is variable. Atrial flutter often presents with a ventricular rate of 150/min, especially in the absence of drug therapy. The heart has a built-in protective mechanism that creates AV nodal block commonly manifested as 2 to 1 AV block so that only every other impulse reaches the ventricles (the only exception is the presence of an accessory pathway).

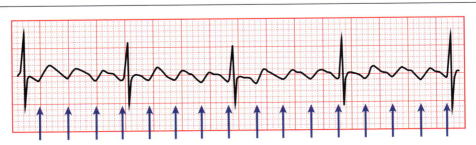

Atrial flutter (with 4:1 AV block) showing with clear inverted flutter waves (arrows). The ventricular rate is 75 - 80/min and the flutter rate is 300/min.

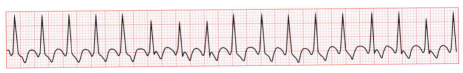

Atrial flutter with 2:1 AV block. The ventricular rate is 150/min. The flutter waves are not seen.

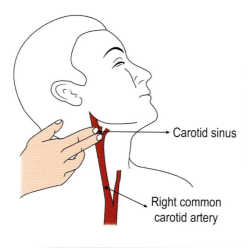

The diagnosis can be corroborated by vagal maneuvers (i.e., carotid sinus massage) and medications which suppress conduction across the AV node so that transient AV block may unmask the flutter waves.

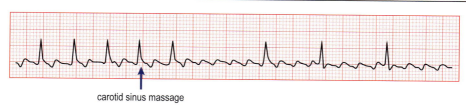

Atrial flutter at a rate of 300/min. Slowing caused by increased delay in AV conduction by carotid sinus massage.

A narrow complex tachycardia at a rate of 150/min should be considered as atrial flutter with 2 to 1 AV block until proven otherwise, especially in the absence of conditions causing sinus tachycardia.

AV Nodal Reentrant Tachycardia

AV nodal reentrant tachycardia (AVNRT) results from a re-entry circuit in or around the AV node.

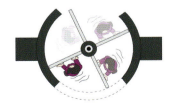

Within the AV node, there exists two functional conduction pathways: the slow pathway (SP) and the fast pathway (FP). Under normal conditions, a regular atrial impulse travels anterogradely through both the SP and FP but the wavefront through the FP is the only one to reach the bundle of His. Conduction over the SP is "blocked" by retrograde invasion of the SP from the wavefront originating in the FP.

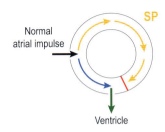

With some individuals, there is an imbalance of the two pathways electrophysiological properties such that an impulse that arrives to the AV node prematurely will conduct down one pathway and up the other creating a continuous loop or reentrant circuit. In AVNRT, an atrial premature impulse finds the FP in a refractory state and conducts down the SP.

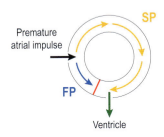

The SP becomes the anterograde limb and the FP, which has recovered from its refractory state, is the retrograde limb of the tachycardia reentry circuit. This is commonly referred to as slow-fast AVNRT. The atria and ventricles are being activated virtually simultaneously from the AV nodal reentrant process.

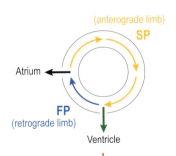

165

The characteristic ECG patterns of AV nodal reentrant tachycardia:

 Regular ventricular rate ranging from 120 - 220/min with narrow QRS complexes unless an intraventricular conduction disturbance is present.

 The P waves are often invisible because they are "hidden" inside the QRS complexes. If seen, they are very close to the QRS complex and inverted in lead II because of retrograde atrial activation.

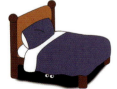

Sometimes, they are "attached" to the QRS complex resulting in a small positive deflection at the end of the QRS complex (pseudo r wave) in lead V1 or a negative deflection at the end of the QRS complex (pseudo S wave) in leads II, III and aVF.

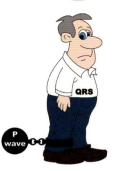

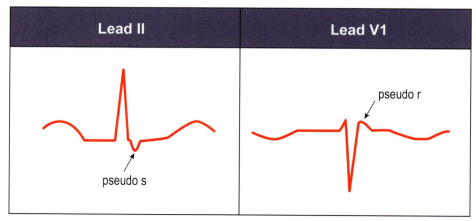

The ECG must be compared to recordings in normal sinus rhythm to establish the diagnosis of the pseudo r and pseudo s deflections by proving the absence of these deflections in normal sinus rhythm.

 Typically, there is 1 to 1 conduction through the AV node. 2 to 1 atrioventricular block occurs rarely.

 Vagal maneuvers may abruptly terminate the tachycardia by slowing AV nodal conduction.

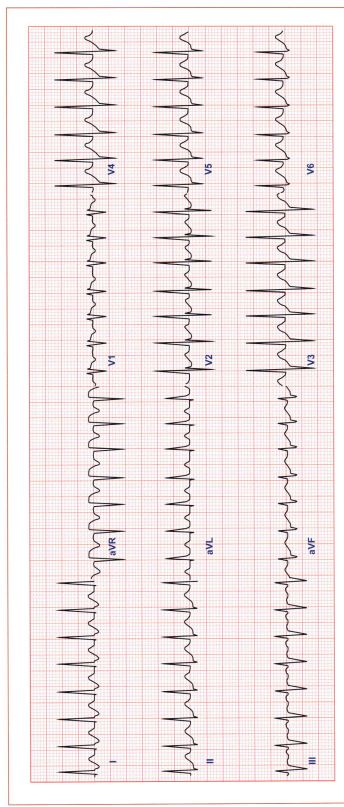

AV nodal reentrant tachycardia with a rapid ventricular rate of 175/min. No clear p waves are seen. The diagnosis was determined during an electrophysiologic study.

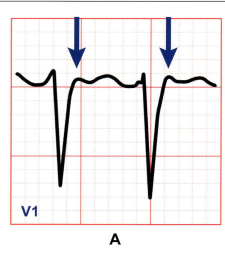 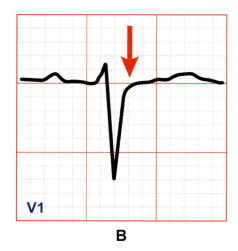

A: AV nodal reentrant tachycardia with pseudo-r waves (blue arrows). The pseudo-r deflections are P waves. B: Normal sinus rhythm with no terminal R wave (red arrow).

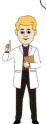

Retrograde P waves are often not visible in AVNRT.

AV Reentrant Tachycardia

AV reentrant tachycardia (AVRT) results from a reentrant circuit involving the AV node and an AV accessory pathway.

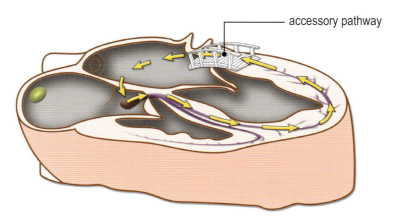

accessory pathway

An accessory pathway is an abnormal small band of myocardial tissue formed during embryogenesis that connects the atria directly with the ventricle. With AVRT, the reentrant circuit is initiated by an impulse that travels through the AV node to the ventricle and then up the accessory pathway back to the atrium.

The characteristic ECG patterns of AV reentrant tachycardia:

1. Regular ventricular rate ranging from 150 – 220/min.

2. Narrow QRS complexes unless there is an intraventricular conduction disturbance.

3. Retrograde P waves which are close but distinct from the QRS complexes (in the ST segment) and inverted in the inferior leads (II, III and aVF). Retrograde atrial activation is more delayed in AVRT compared to AVNRT because the impulse has to travel through the ventricle to reach the accessory pathway.

4. Vagal maneuvers may abruptly terminate the tachycardia by slowing AV nodal conduction.

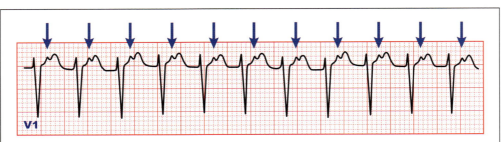

AV reentrant tachycardia with a ventricular rate of 165/min. Retrograde P waves are clearly seen after the QRS complex on the ST segment (arrows).

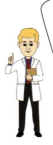

Vagal maneuvers will either terminate or have no effect on AVRT or AVNRT. In contrast, atrial flutter will not terminate but may exhibit varying degrees of AV block.

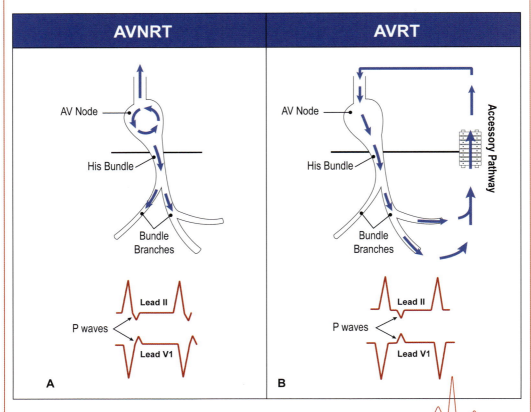

170

Sick Sinus Syndrome

Sick sinus syndrome is characterized by sinus bradyarrhythmias (sinus bradycardia, sinus arrest or sinoatrial exit block) and may be accompanied by paroxysmal supraventricular tachyarrhythmias. Atrial fibrillation is the most common tachyarrhythmia, but atrial flutter and atrial tachycardia can also occur. The alternation of bradycardia and tachycardia is commonly known as bradycardia-tachycardia syndrome (or brady-tachy syndrome). In this syndrome, abrupt termination of tachycardia can be accompanied by a relatively long period of asystole (both atrial and ventricular) with no sinus or other "rescue" activity. This is called overdrive suppression. The absence of a rapidly emerging escape rhythm after tachycardia termination indicates that sick sinus syndrome also affects the AV junction.

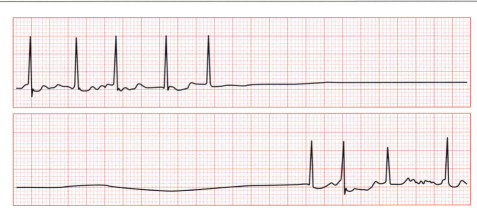

Bradycardia-tachycardia syndrome. Atrial fibrillation followed by a long period of asystole of 6 seconds and attempted termination.

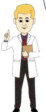

Bradycardia-tachycardia syndrome form of sick sinus syndrome is a diffuse disease involving the atrium and the conduction system. Termination of intermittent tachycardia may cause ventricular asystole by overdrive suppression.

171

Evaluation of a Narrow QRS Complex Tachycardia

 Determine regularity

Regular Rhythm	Irregular Rhythm
• Sinus tachycardia • Atrial flutter • Atrial tachycardia • AVNRT • AVRT • Junctional tachycardia	• Atrial fibrillation • Atrial flutter with varying AV block • Atrial tachycardia with varying AV block • Multifocal atrial tachycardia

 If P waves are visible

 What is the direction (upright or inverted) of the P waves?

P waves that are inverted in leads II, III and aVF are "retrograde" P waves. Retrograde P waves can be seen with a junctional tachycardia, AVNRT and AVRT.

Where are they in relation to the QRS complex (before, after, or "attached")?

P waves that closely follow the QRS complexes suggests AVRT. Distinct P waves before and close to the QRS complex suggests sinus tachycardia or focal atrial tachycardia. P waves that are "attached" to the QRS complexes (pseudo r' wave in lead V1 or pseudo S wave in leads II, III and aVF) suggests AVNRT.

Are there more P waves than QRS complexes?

More P waves than QRS complexes suggests atrial flutter or atrial tachycardia with AV block and essentially rules out a tachycardia involving the AV node as a reentrant loop (AVNRT, AVRT). Often, the fast atrial rate associated with atrial flutter (commonly 300/min) is not clearly visible because a 2 to 1 AV block is present.

3. Response to vagal maneuvers or medications to slow AV nodal conduction

Vagal maneuvers or medications will either terminate or have no effect on AVNRT or AVRT. On the other hand, they may unmask atrial flutter, atrial fibrillation or atrial tachycardia.

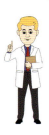

Atrial flutter with 2:1 block and atrial tachycardia are often mistaken for sinus tachycardia. Keep in mind that sinus tachycardia rarely exceeds a heart rate more than 140/min unless the patient is extremely sick.

Wolf Parkinson White Syndrome

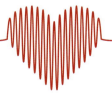

Wolf Parkinson White Syndrome

Wolf Parkinson White syndrome (WPW) is characterized by a ventricular preexcitation pattern resulting from an abnormal accessory pathway connecting the atrium directly to the ventricle.

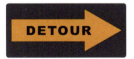

The characteristic ECG patterns of Wolf Parkinson White syndrome:

1. The PR interval is short (< 0.12 sec).

2. There is slurred upstroke of the QRS complex referred to as a delta wave.

3. The QRS complex is > 0.11 sec.

4. There are secondary ST-T wave changes.

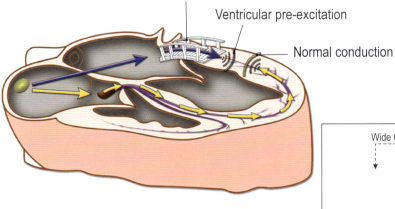

175

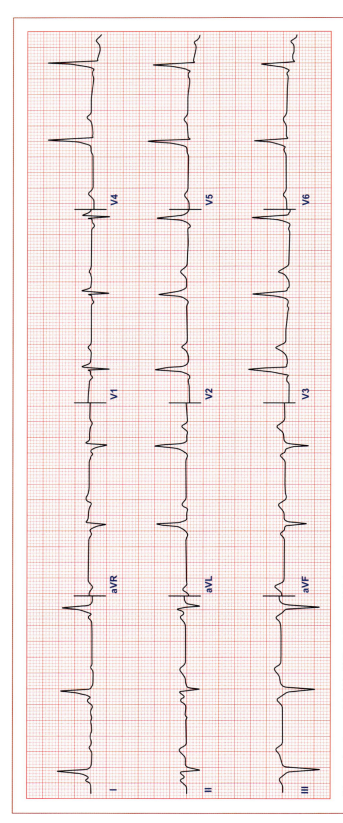

Sinus rhythm with Wolf Parkinson White syndrome. The PR intervals are short and the QRS complexes are wide (> 0.11 sec) with slurred upstroke (delta waves). Note the Q waves in leads III and aVF. Q waves can sometimes be seen with WPW if the accessory pathway is in a specific location.

Wolf Parkinson White syndrome (WPW) may be associated with supraventricular tachyarrhythmias including reentrant tachycardias and atrial fibrillation. Orthodromic Atrioventricular Reentry Tachycardia (AVRT) is the most common form of reentrant tachycardia and involves anterograde conduction (atria —> ventricle) via the AV node and retrograde conduction (ventricle —> atria) via the accessory pathway. Consequently, the characteristic wide QRS complex and delta wave are not visible. Rarely, when the circuit is activated in the opposite direction, antidromic AVRT will supervene with a wide QRS complex of pre-excitation.

Wolf Parkinson White syndrome with AVRT

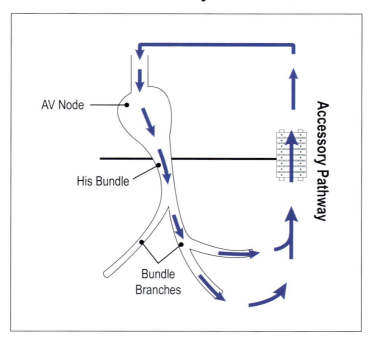

If atrial fibrillation develops, the normal rate limiting or braking effect of the AV node is bypassed. This allows the atrial impulses to activate the ventricles partially or completely via the accessory pathway.

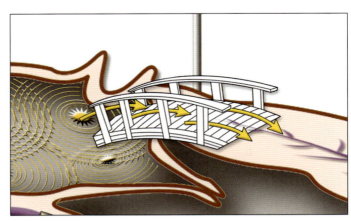

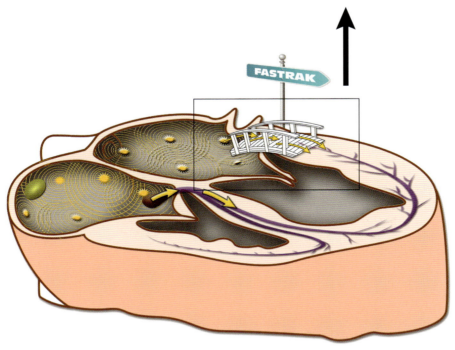

The characteristic ECG patterns of atrial fibrillation associated with WPW:

 An irregularly irregular rhythm.

 Ventricular rate may reach 250-300 /min. Such rates cannot occur in a normal heart.

 Intermittent or persistently wide QRS complexes. The QRS pattern may be quite variable in terms of morphology and RR interval and will depend on how much in any given cycle the ventricle is depolarized via the AV node or the accessory pathway. The QRS complexes can sometimes vary from cycle to cycle and may be narrow, wide or intermediate (fusion beats*). This may create a confusing ECG resembling polymorphic ventricular tachycardia*.

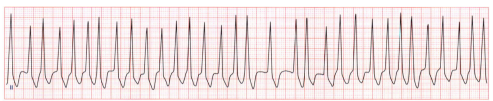

The average HR is 200/min. Some of the RR intervals are 0.2 seconds and representative of a malignant form of WPW susceptible to extremely fast ventricular rates.

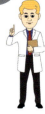

Atrial fibrillation with WPW can be mistaken for polymorphic ventricular tachycardia. An irregular wide QRS tachycardia with a ventricular rate > 200/min should raise suspicion for atrial fibrillation with an accessory pathway.

Fusion beats and polymorphic ventricular tachycardia are discussed in the ventricular arrhythmia and ventricular tachyarrhythmia sections.

Ventricular Arrhythmias

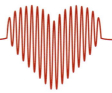

Ventricular Premature Complexes

A ventricular premature complex (VPC) is the result of premature ventricular activation from an impulse originating from a ventricular ectopic focus. A ventricular premature impulse does not engage the His-Purkinje conduction system. Instead, conduction occurs via the ordinary myocardium which conducts more slowly.

A ventricular premature impulse often results in retrograde conduction into and activation of the AV node, but the impulse rarely travels as far as the atrium.

The characteristic ECG patterns of a ventricular premature complex:

1. Wide QRS complex (≥ 0.12 sec).

2. Bizarre appearing QRS complex.

3. Absence of a P wave preceding the QRS complex.

4. The ST segment and T wave are opposite in direction to the main direction of the QRS.

5. Usually, a ventricular premature impulse fails to conduct retrogradely to the atrium because of functional AV block. The SA node continues to fire normally. However, the next sinus P wave is often not visible and conduction of the atrial impulse through the AV node is blocked because of refractoriness created by the VPC. As a result, the PP interval encompassing the VPC (from the P wave before the VPC to the next conducted P wave after the VPC) measures twice the prevailing sinus PP interval. This ECG pattern is referred to as a "VPC with a compensatory pause". (Note: Double the PP interval doubles the RR interval provided the PR is constant).

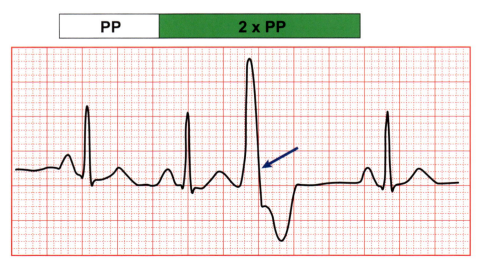

Sinus rhythm with a ventricular premature complex (arrow). The QRS of the VPC is wide and is not preceded by a P wave. The PP interval encompassing the VPC (green bar) is exactly double the prevailing sinus PP interval (white bar). The RR interval encompassing the VPC also measures double the prevailing RR interval since the PR intervals are constant.

The PP interval encompassing the ventricular premature complex is usually double the prevailing sinus PP interval. This indicates a "compensatory pause" which does not occur with atrial premature complexes with rare exceptions.

Sometimes, but not often, a VPC is not followed by a pause. This is referred to as an "interpolated" VPC. The SA node continues to fire normally and anterograde conduction through the AV node is maintained resulting in a VPC that is sandwiched between two normally conducted sinus beats.

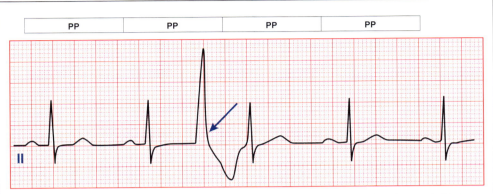

Sinus rhythm with an interpolated ventricular premature complex (arrow). Note the absence of a pause after the VPC.

 An APC with aberrancy may be similar in appearance to a VPC. A VPC is not preceded by a P wave and is often associated with a "compensatory pause".

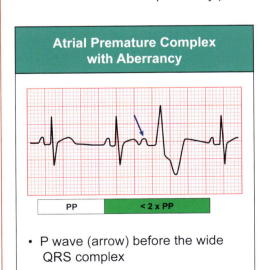

Atrial Premature Complex with Aberrancy

- P wave (arrow) before the wide QRS complex
- "Non-compensatory pause"

Ventricular Premature Complex

- P wave absent before the wide QRS complex
- "Compensatory pause"

183

Ventricular premature complexes can be classified as follows:

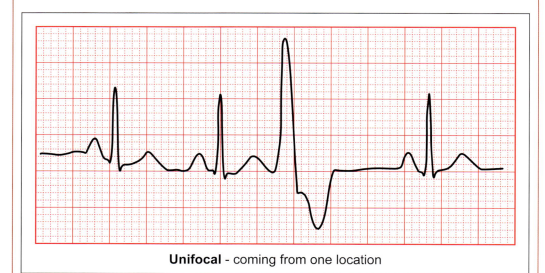

Unifocal - coming from one location

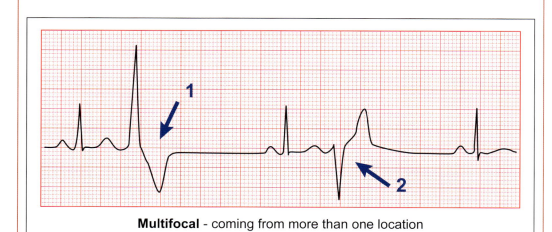

Multifocal - coming from more than one location

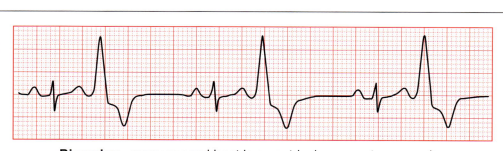

Bigeminy - every second beat is a ventricular premature complex

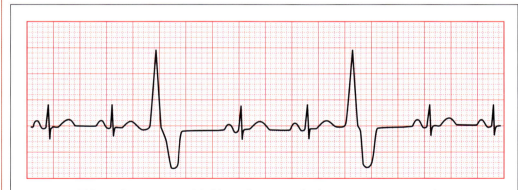

Trigeminy - every third beat is a ventricular premature complex

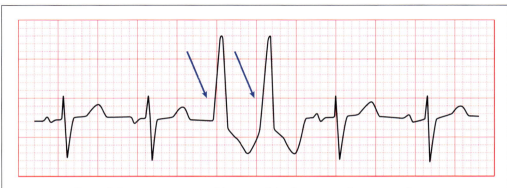

Couplet - a sequence of two ventricular premature complexes

A sequence of three ventricular premature complexes is often referred to as a triplet. By definition, three or more successive ventricular complexes at a rate of > 100/min is considered ventricular tachycardia (covered under Ventricular Tachyarrhythmias).

Ventricular Escape Rhythm

A ventricular escape rhythm occurs when the ventricles take over as the primary pacemaker of the heart because of the inability of the sinus and/or AV junction to generate a take-over impulse.

The characteristic ECG patterns of a ventricular escape rhythm:

 Ventricular rate ≤ 45/min.

 Wide QRS complexes (≥ 0.12 sec).

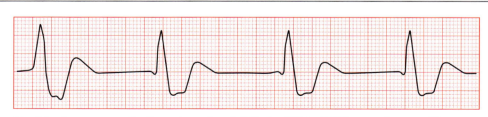

Ventricular escape rhythm at a rate of 42/min. Wide QRS complexes with no visible P waves.

Accelerated Idioventricular Rhythm

Accelerated idioventricular rhythm (AIVR) is an enhanced ectopic ventricular rhythm that is generally transient and often occurs after a myocardial infarction.

The characteristic ECG patterns of an accelerated idioventricular rhythm (AIVR):

 There must be at least three consecutive ventricular complexes (QRS ≥ 0.12 sec) and a rate between 60-100/min.

 There are frequently fusion beats at the onset and termination of this rhythm. Fusion beats are the result of activation of the ventricles from two depolarization fronts, one originating from the sinoatrial node and the other from the ectopic focus in the ventricle.

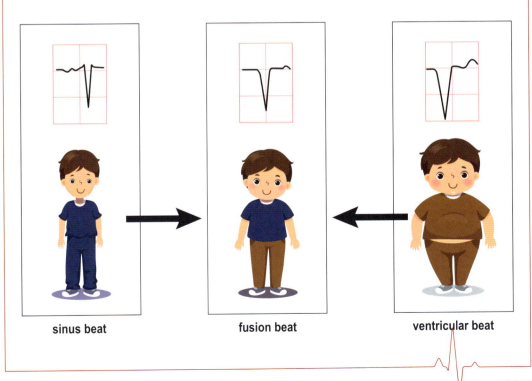

187

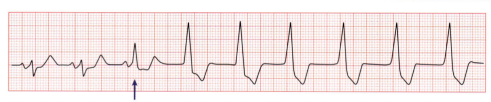

Onset of accelerated idioventricular rhythm. Note the fusion beat (arrow) sandwiched between the sinus beats and the start of the accelerated idioventricular rhythm.

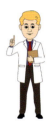

At first glance, accelerated idioventricular rhythm may appear to be a bundle branch block. With accelerated idioventricular rhythm, there are no P waves in front of the QRS complexes as in sinus rhythm.

Ventricular Tachyarrhythmias

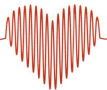

Ventricular Tachycardia

Ventricular tachycardia (VT) is an ectopic ventricular rhythm defined as three or more successive ventricular complexes at a rate of >100/min. The most common cause of ventricular tachycardia is post-myocardial infarction. Ventricular tachycardia can be classified by type and duration.

- **Duration** -   sustained (lasting > 30 seconds) vs unsustained (< 30 seconds)

- **Type** -   monomorphic (stable and uniform in morphology) vs polymorphic (unstable and irregular in morphology and rate)

Monomorphic Ventricular Tachycardia

The characteristic ECG patterns of monomorphic ventricular tachycardia:

1 Stable and uniform QRS complexes ≥ 0.12 sec.

2 The rhythm is usually regular, although slight irregularity can occur.

3 There are a few other features of monomorphic ventricular tachycardia but they are commonly not present on the ECG (important - their absence in **NO WAY** rules out ventricular tachycardia).

a Fusion beats — confirms the diagnosis of ventricular tachycardia in the setting of a regular wide QRS complex tachycardia.

b AV Dissociation — If present, it is diagnostic of ventricular tachycardia. Although not uncommon, its ECG footprint is rarely seen because the P waves are often not discernible.

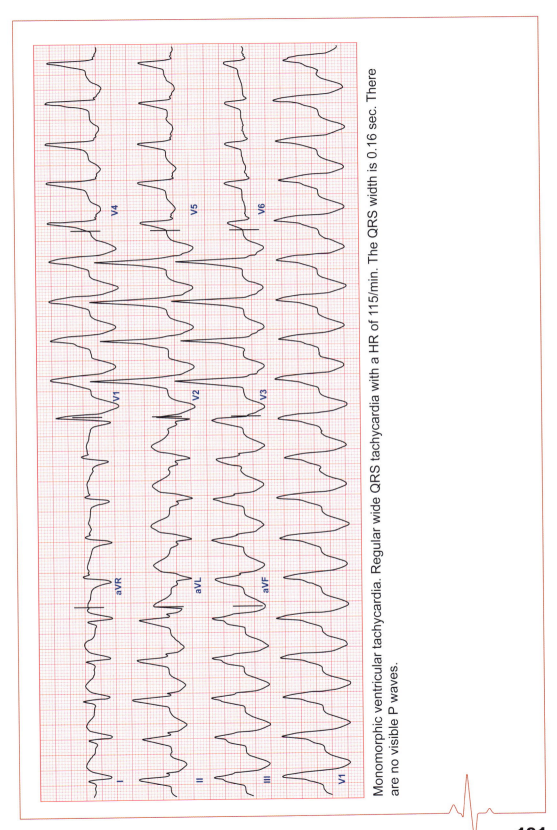

Monomorphic ventricular tachycardia. Regular wide QRS tachycardia with a HR of 115/min. The QRS width is 0.16 sec. There are no visible P waves.

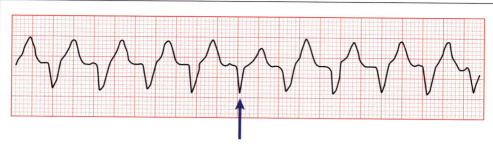

Ventricular tachycardia at a rate of 125 - 135/min. The fifth complex (arrow) represents a fusion beat which occurs when the ventricles are activated by both a sinus impulse and an impulse from the ventricular ectopic focus. Fusion beats in a wide QRS complex tachycardia makes the diagnosis of ventricular tachycardia.

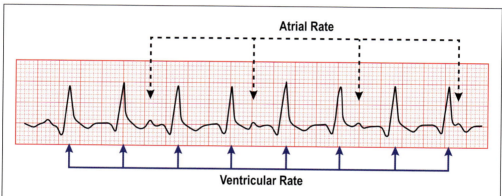

Ventricular tachycardia with AV dissociation. The ventricular rate (120/min) is faster than the atrial rate (62/min). AV dissociation in the setting of a regular wide QRS complex tachycardia is diagnostic of ventricular tachycardia.

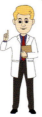

Fusion beats and AV dissociation are uncommonly seen on the ECG and their absence in no way rules out ventricular tachycardia.

Torsades de Pointes

Polymorphic ventricular tachycardia is less common than monomorphic ventricular tachycardia, is dangerous and often a precursor to ventricular fibrillation. Torsades de Pointes ("twisting of the points") is a specific form of polymorphic ventricular tachycardia and associated with long QT syndrome.

The characteristic ECG patterns of Torsades de Pointes:

1 Sinusoidal alteration of the QRS axis with rotation of the electrical axis by 180° every 5-20 beats.

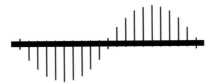

2 Wide QRS complexes (≥ 0.12 sec) with varying configuration and varying RR intervals.

3 Ventricular rate of 160-250/min.

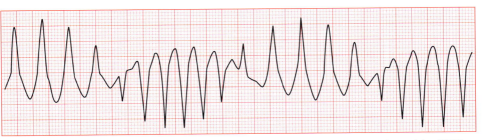

Torsades de Pointes (twisting of the points). There is rapid, irregular wide QRS complexes with twisting of the QRS axis every 5-6 beats.

Long QT Syndrome

Long QT syndrome is a disorder characterized by prolongation of the QT interval (QTc > 0.46 sec in men and > 0.44 sec in women) on the basic ECG. Acquired causes of a long QT include medications such as antibiotics, antipsychotics, and antiarrhythmics as well as electrolyte imbalances. Long QT syndrome may also be congenital.

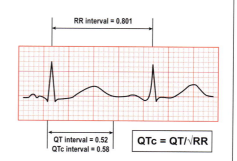

Prolonged QTc interval

Wide QRS Complex Tachycardia

A wide QRS complex tachycardia is defined as a rhythm on the ECG with a HR > 100/min and QRS duration ≥ 0.12 sec. A wide complex tachycardia can be ventricular or supraventricular in origin. Ventricular tachycardia (VT) is by far the most common cause of a wide complex tachycardia and carries the worst prognosis. Supraventricular tachyarrhythmia with a pre-existing bundle branch block (SVT with aberrancy) is the second commonest cause.

Differentiating between VT and SVT with aberrancy on the ECG can be very challenging. Wide complex tachycardias are often incorrectly diagnosed as SVT with aberrancy and treatment of ventricular tachycardia for SVT with aberrancy may result in potentially disastrous consequences. A variety of algorithms to differentiate ventricular tachycardia from supraventricular tachycardia with aberrancy have been proposed, however, they are complex and not always reliable. For these reasons, the following rules should apply.

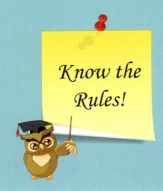

RULE #1 - Treat a regular wide QRS complex tachycardia as ventricular tachycardia until proven otherwise.

RULE #2 - A regular wide QRS complex tachycardia in a patient with known heart disease almost always indicates ventricular tachycardia.

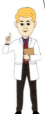

Fast, regular and wide is VT until proven otherwise!

Ventricular Flutter

Ventricular flutter is a form of very rapid regular monomorphic ventricular tachycardia that often deteriorates into ventricular fibrillation. The rate is usually 300/min. The ECG looks the same when it is visualized upside-down.

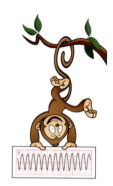

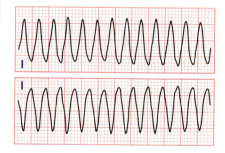

Top: Ventricular flutter with a ventricular rate of about 300/min. **Bottom**: The same ECG is turned upside-down and looks similar.

Ventricular Fibrillation

With ventricular fibrillation (VF), there is total chaos in the ventricles. There are numerous micro-reentrant circuits occurring within the ventricles at the same time. This results in multiple attempted or partial QRS complexes of varying morphology and height. Coordinated ventricular activity is impossible.

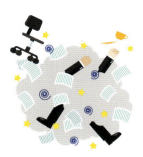

The characteristic ECG patterns of ventricular fibrillation:

1 There are no discernible P waves, ST segments or T waves.

2 Instead of seeing the typical QRS complexes, there are ventricular fibrillary waves which occur at a frequency of 350 – 450/min.

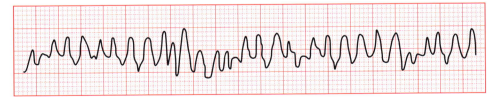

Ventricular fibrillation. Rapid (HR > 300/min) grossly irregular ventricular rhythm with no identifiable P waves, QRS complexes or T waves. The fibrillatory waves vary in shape, timing and amplitude.

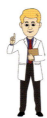

An ECG that resembles the disorganized activity of ventricular fibrillation may be generated by artifact.

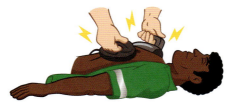

If no intervention occurs within minutes, ventricular fibrillation degenerates into asystole (absence of any discernible rhythm on ECG or flat line) and death.

Atrioventricular Conduction Blocks

Atrioventricular (AV) conduction blocks involve a disturbance in conduction of the cardiac impulse between the atria and ventricles. The conduction disturbance can vary from a mild delay to a complete "block".

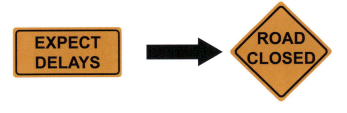
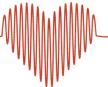

First Degree AV Block

The term "block" in electrocardiography describes a delay in conduction or a true conduction block. First degree AV block is a conduction delay and often occurs at the AV node but can occur anywhere between the atria and ventricles.

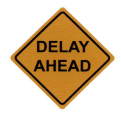

The characteristic ECG patterns of first degree AV block:

 PR interval is > 0.21 sec.

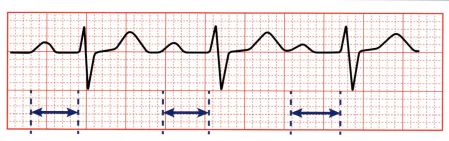

Sinus rhythm with first degree AV block. The PR intervals (arrows) are 0.24 sec.

First degree AV block is a delay, not a true block.

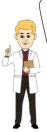

If the delay is marked, the P wave may be concealed by the preceding T wave.

Second Degree AV Block

With second degree AV block, there is impaired conduction of the atrial impulse within the AV node or His-Purkinje system resulting in intermittent "non-conducted" P waves (P waves not followed by a QRS complex). These "non-conducted" P waves are often referred to as "blocked" P waves. There are currently four types of second degree AV block.

1. Type I Second Degree AV Block

2. Type II Second Degree AV Block

3. 2:1 Second Degree AV Block

4. Advanced Second Degree AV Block

Type I Second Degree AV Block

Type I second degree AV block, also referred to as Mobitz type I or Wenckebach type I AV block, involves the occurrence in sinus rhythm of a "non-conducted" P wave associated with **inconstant** PR intervals before and after the blocked impulse.

The ECG features of type I second degree AV block:

Type I second degree AV block can be described in terms of the "classic" (traditional) form or the "atypical" form.

"Classic" Form - associated with progressive prolongation of the PR intervals culminating with a single "non-conducted" sinus P wave. The second PR interval always shows the greatest increment of conduction.

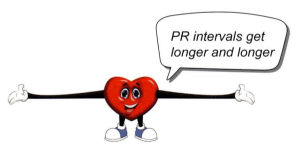

PR intervals get longer and longer

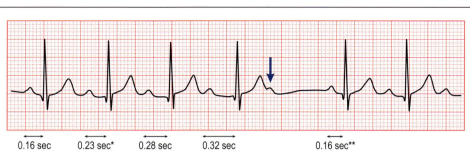

0.16 sec   0.23 sec*   0.28 sec   0.32 sec   0.16 sec**

Sinus rhythm with "classic" type I second degree AV block. There is progressive prolongation of the PR intervals followed by a "non-conducted" P wave (blue arrow). The second PR interval (*) shows the greatest increment of conduction. There is shortening of the PR interval of the conducted beat after the "non-conducted" P wave (**).

"Atypical" Form - 50% or more of type I sequences do not conform to the "classic" pattern and are characterized by a single P wave preceded by gradual but irregular PR prolongation with occasional unpredictable changes anywhere within a conducted sequence. The PR intervals may stabilize and show no evidence of prolongation in the middle or for several beats at the end of a type I sequence.

 The diagnosis **requires** the presence of sinus rhythm and at least 2 consecutively conducted P waves before the "block" of a single P wave.

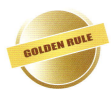

At least 3 P's to 2 QRS's before the block must be present before a diagnose of type I can be made

 The hallmark of all forms of type I second degree AV block is shortening of the PR interval after the "blocked" P wave. This fact is of utmost importance in the differentiation of type I block from type II block (covered in the next section).

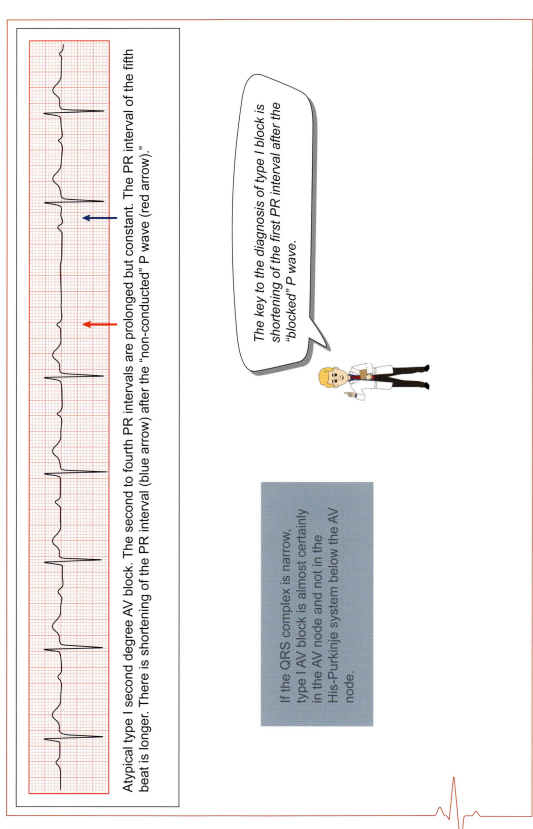

Type II Second Degree AV Block

Type II second degree AV block, also referred to as Mobitz type II AV block, involves the occurrence in sinus rhythm of a single "non-conducted" P wave associated with **constant** PR intervals before and after the blocked impulse.

The ECG features of type II second degree AV block:

1 The diagnosis **requires** the presence of sinus rhythm and at least 2 consecutively conducted P waves before the "block" of a single P wave.

2 All of the PR intervals must remain constant before and after the "blocked" P wave to make the diagnosis of type II AV block. The hallmark of the diagnosis is an unchanged PR interval after the "blocked" P wave.

3 To make this diagnosis, the sinus rate must be regular with no evidence of transient sinus slowing (increase in PP interval). Simultaneous sinus slowing and AV nodal block from a vagal surge can produce an ECG pattern that resembles type II second degree AV block.

4 Another signature of type II second degree AV block is based on the constancy of the sinus rate so that the RR interval encompassing the "blocked" P wave is twice as long as the previous RR interval.

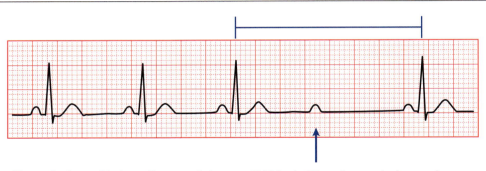

Sinus rhythm with type II second degree AV block. The sinus rate is regular. The PR intervals before and after the "non-conducted" P wave (blue arrow) are constant. The RR interval encompassing the block (blue interval) is twice that of the RR interval prior to the "non-conducted" P wave.

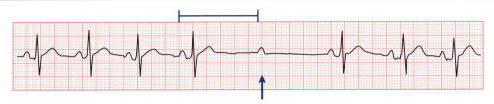

Vagal induced AV block. There is sinus slowing as evident by the increase in the PP interval (blue interval) prior to the "non-conducted" P wave (blue arrow). The diagnosis of type II second degree AV block cannot be considered when there is sinus slowing.

> The QRS complex is often wide but may occasionally be narrow. Properly defined type II second degree AV block is always serious as it involves the His-Purkinje system.

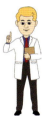

The diagnosis of type II AV block cannot be made in the absence of an unchanged PR interval after the "blocked" P wave.

2:1 Second Degree AV Block

The ECG features of 2:1 second degree AV block:

 Every alternate P wave is "blocked".

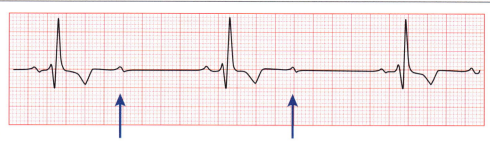

Sinus rhythm with 2:1 second degree AV block. Every other P wave is "blocked" (blue arrows). The QRS is wide. This is neither type I nor type II second degree AV block.

A very common mistake in electrocardiography labels 2:1 AV block either as type I or type II AV block.

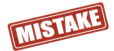

> 2:1 second degree AV block is neither type I nor type II AV block.
> **It is simply 2:1 AV block.**

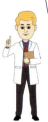

2:1 block is neither type I nor type II.

Advanced Second Degree AV Block

Advanced second degree AV block includes 3:1, 4:1 or higher. 3:1 means three P waves for each QRS complex. This form of block cannot be classified in terms of type I and type II second degree AV blocks.

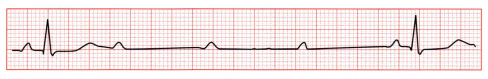

Advanced second degree AV block with a blocking ratio of 4:1.

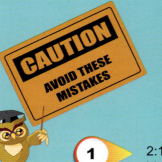

Pitfalls In The Diagnosis of Type II Second Degree AV Block

1 2:1 AV block may be misdiagnosed as type II AV block.

2 Misdiagnosis of type II AV block remains common in the setting of transient sinus slowing from a vagal surge. The diagnosis of type II AV block should not be made if there is any slowing of the sinus rate.

3 Type I AV block may be misdiagnosed as type II AV block when the last two or more PR intervals before the block are constant. Additionally, failure to notice shortening of the PR interval after the block.

4 A blocked atrial premature complex may superficially resemble type II AV block. The difference is that the atrial premature complex is early but the sinus rhythm is constant and regular in type II AV block.

Third Degree AV Block

In third degree heart block (or complete heart block), none of the cardiac impulses from the atria are conducted to the ventricles. The atria and the ventricles are activated independently of each other.

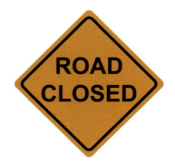

The ECG features of third degree AV block:

1. Sinus P waves "march" right through showing no association with the QRS complexes.

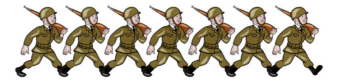

2. Evidence of a slower junctional or ventricular escape rhythm.

3. Atrial rate > ventricular rate. This is the hallmark of complete heart block and ignoring this simple concept will lead to diagnostic errors.

4. The QRS may be narrow or wide depending on the origin of the escape rhythm.

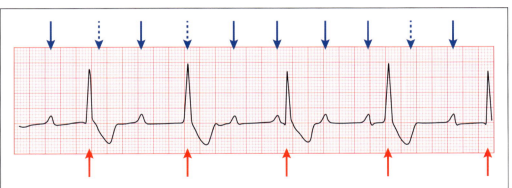

Third degree AV block. The P waves do not bear any relationship with the QRS complexes. The atrial rate (blue arrows) is faster than the ventricular rate (red arrows).

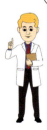

With third degree AV block, the key to the diagnosis is that the atrial rate is faster than the ventricular rate.

AV Dissociation

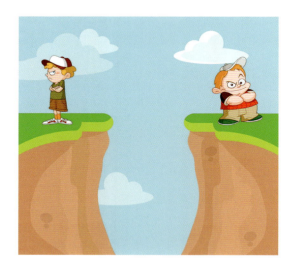

Atrioventricular dissociation is an electrocardiographic manifestation of independent activity of the atria and ventricles. It is the result of an arrhythmia, not an arrhythmia itself.

Atrioventricular dissociation may be seen with the following arrhythmias:

1 Third degree (complete) AV block.

2 A junctional or ventricular escape rhythm when the sinus node has failed.

3 A junctional or ventricular rhythm which takes over control of the heart rate (accelerated junctional rhythm, junctional tachycardia, accelerated idioventricular ventricular rhythm or ventricular tachycardia). Normal AV conduction resumes after the arrhythmia.

> The ECG shows sinus P waves that bear no relation to the QRS complexes. The P waves "march through" the QRS complexes.

The key to sorting out the underlying arrhythmia is measuring the atrial rate and the ventricular rate. If the atrial rate is faster than the ventricular rate, there is underlying third degree (complete) heart block. In the presence of a junctional or ventricular rhythm, the ventricular rate is faster than the atrial rate.

Third degree AV block is often wrongly defined as AV dissociation. The latter is a symptom not a diagnosis.

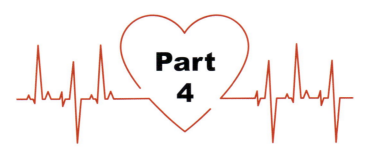

Miscellaneous Abnormalities

Hyperkalemia

There are a number of ECG abnormalities seen with hyperkalemia (K > 5.2 mEq/L) and these findings generally correlate with the potassium level. However, life threatening arrhythmias have been reported at different levels of hyperkalemia which may be the result of underlying cardiac pathology. A serum potassium of 5.5 - 6.5 mEq/L may be associated with peaked T waves seen most commonly in the precordial leads. A serum level of 6.6 - 8.0 mEq/L may be associated with widening and flattening of the P wave, prolonged PR interval, high grade AV block with slow junctional or ventricular escape rhythm, intraventricular conduction disturbances and progressive widening of the QRS complex and eventual merging with the T wave to form a sine wave.

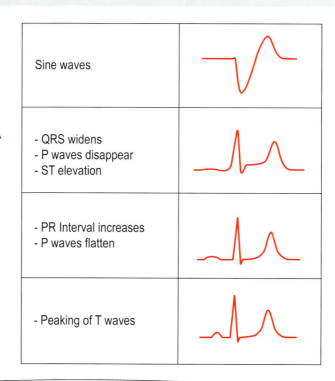

increasing potassium level (hyperkalemia)

Sine waves	
- QRS widens - P waves disappear - ST elevation	
- PR Interval increases - P waves flatten	
- Peaking of T waves	

Hyperkalemia should be ruled out in the presence of an idioventricular rhythm with no visible P waves and a very broad QRS > 0.2 sec.

Hypokalemia

ECG abnormalities associated with hypokalemia (K < 3.5 mEq/L) may include ST segment depression, shallow T wave and a prominent U wave. The U wave is a small deflection immediately following the T wave that is often not visualized on the normal ECG, however, can be prominent with hypokalemia.

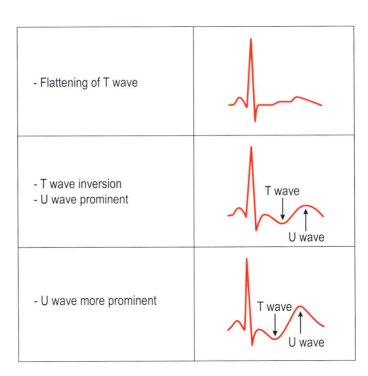

Pulmonary Embolism

A number of findings may be seen in the presence of a pulmonary embolism, however, none of them are very sensitive or specific.

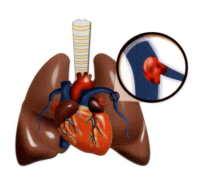

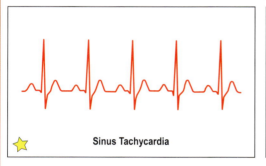

⭐ Sinus Tachycardia

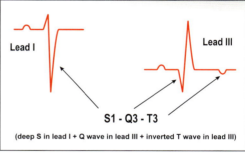

S1 - Q3 - T3
(deep S in lead I + Q wave in lead III + inverted T wave in lead III)

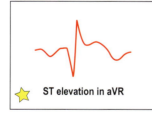

⭐ ST elevation in aVR

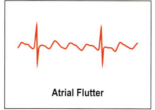

Atrial Flutter

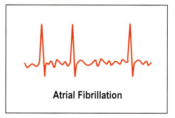

Atrial Fibrillation

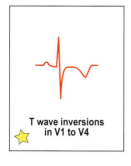

⭐ T wave inversions in V1 to V4

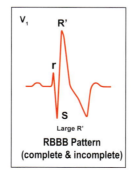

RBBB Pattern
(complete & incomplete)

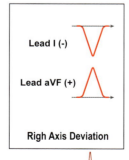

Righ Axis Deviation

⭐ *Most common*

Low Voltage

Low voltage is usually defined as a QRS amplitude of < 10 mm (10 small boxes) in the precordial leads and < 5 mm (5 small boxes) in the limb leads. This finding is associated with various conditions including a cardiomyopathy, congestive heart failure, a pericardial effusion, obesity, chronic obstructive lung disease, a pneumothorax and an infiltrative process involving the heart.

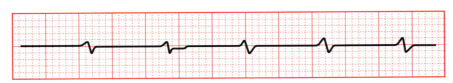

QRS amplitude in frontal leads (I, II, III, aVR, aVL, and aVF) < 5mm

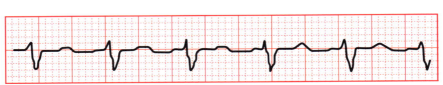

QRS amplitude in precordial leads (V1 to V6) < 10 mm

Electrical Alternans

Electrical alternans is an alternation of the QRS complex amplitude or axis between cycles. This is seen with severe pericardial effusion and cardiac tamponade (build up of fluid in the pericardial sac resulting in compression of the heart).

Normal Heart   **Pericardial Effusion**

Pericardium   Buildup of fluid

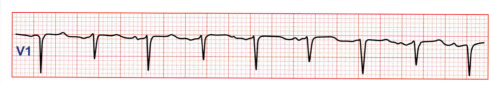

Electrical alternans. There is alternating amplitude of the QRS complexes. This finding is most commonly associated with a large pericardial effusion.

Pacemaker

An electronic pacemaker is a device that is surgically implanted to regulate the heart beat in the setting of severe heart rhythm disturbances such as AV blocks or sick sinus syndrome. Pacing systems consist of two parts: a battery-operated pulse generator and one or more intracardiac leads (wires). Pacemakers work on demand which means that they only pace when the heart rate falls below a predetermined level. Single chamber (univentricular) pacemakers use a single right ventricular lead. Dual chamber pacemakers have both atrial and ventricular leads which helps maintain AV synchrony and also prevent some of the limitations of univentricular pacers.

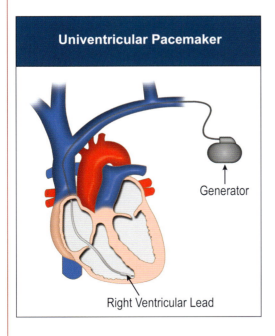

Univentricular Pacemaker

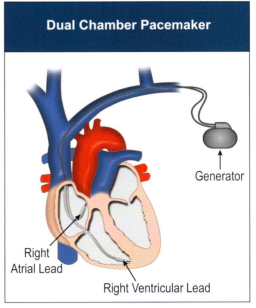

Dual Chamber Pacemaker

There are two basic functions of a demand pacemaker: sensing spontaneous electrical activity and pacing (firing) if needed. When a pacemaker fires, a small spike is seen on the ECG before the P wave and/or QRS complex depending on the type of pacemaker. Pacing in the right ventricle generates a wide and bizarre QRS complex and an ECG similar to a left bundle branch block pattern with similar ST-T wave abnormalities. A paced rhythm can therefore mask certain electrocardiographic abnormalities, including myocardial infarction. With atrial pacing, the paced P wave can be small and not clearly discernible.

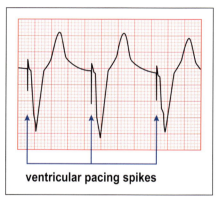

ventricular pacing spikes

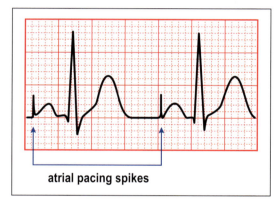

atrial pacing spikes

Paced spikes look like vertical signals but not always obvious. Look carefully in each ECG lead to make sure you're not missing a subtle paced spike!

The timing function of a simple univentricular pacemaker provides the framework for all pacemakers. The programmed pacemaker (PM) interval refers to the lowest rate the pacemaker will pace.

If the programmed PM interval elapses without evidence of ventricular activity, the pacemaker will deliver a stimulus which restarts its own programmed interval by resetting the pacemaker.

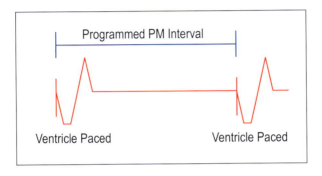

If ventricular activity is sensed before the programmed interval of the pacemaker has elapsed, the pacemaker inhibits release of pacing and restarts its programmed interval pacemaker clock.

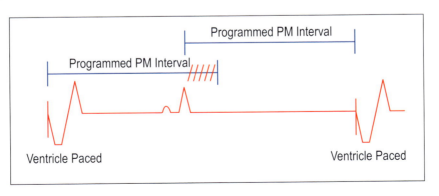

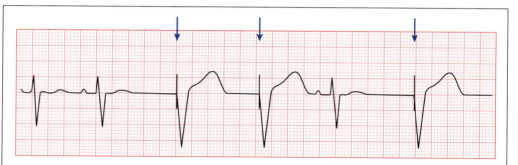

Single chamber right ventricular pacing with normal capture and sensing. The pacemaker fires if it detects no spontaneous activity at the end of the set automatic interval that corresponds to the programmed rate. The 3rd, 4th and 6th complexes are paced beats as indicated by the preceding pacer spike (blue arrows). The pacemaker adequately senses the 1st, 2nd and 5th complexes which are sinus beats.

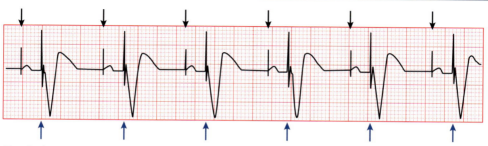

Dual chamber pacing at rest. Note the pacing stimuli (spikes) before the P waves (black arrows) and before the QRS complexes (blue arrows).

Dual chamber pacemakers are designed to maintain AV synchrony during effort or exercise.

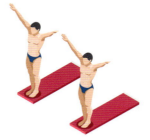

In individuals with normal sinus function and the ability to increase their sinus rate on exercise, the pacemaker will track (sense) the spontaneous P wave and then deliver a ventricular pacing stimulus after a delay. Hence, the name P-synchronous pacing. After the PM senses the P wave, there is a delay before pacing of the ventricle in order to mimic normal AV synchrony (PR interval). The ventricular pacing rate will increase on exercise according to the atrial rate. For safety, these pacemakers have an upper rate limit for ventricular pacing to prevent a dangerous ventricular rate during a rapid atrial tachycardia.

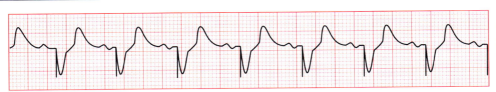

Dual chamber pacing on exercise. The pacing rate has increased to 90 per min. The atrial lead of the pacemaker tracks the P wave so that it can deliver ventricular pacing after a short interval corresponding to the PR interval.

Dual chamber pacemakers are designed with special sensors to detect motion with exercise and translate the signals into an increase of pacing rate if there is inadequate atrial response from underlying sinus node dysfunction (i.e. sick sinus syndrome). This way, AV synchrony is maintained. Single chamber pacemakers can also be sensor driven.

Sometimes, univentricular pacemakers are not able to perform their intended function.

Here are a few common causes of univentricular pacemaker malfunction and their associated ECG findings:

Out of Order!

Failure to capture — the ventricle fails to respond to the pacemaker impulse. On an ECG tracing, the pacemaker spike will appear but will not be followed by a QRS complex.

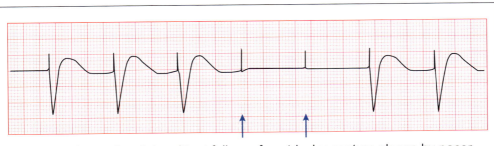

Univentricular pacing. Intermittent failure of ventricular capture shown by pacer stimuli not followed by a QRS complex (arrows).

Failure to sense (undersensing) — the pacemaker does not detect myocardial depolarization. This can often be seen on an ECG tracing as a spike too early after the QRS complex.

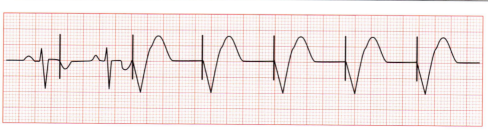

Univentricular pacing. Ventricular undersensing. The first two ventricular complexes are not sensed by the device. The pacemaker captures the ventricle after the second ventricular complex. The first stimuli is ineffective because it falls in the myocardial refractory period.

 Failure to fire — there are intervals longer than the programmed pacer interval with missing pacemaker stimuli.

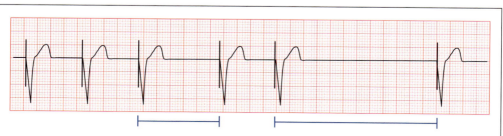

Univentricular pacing. Pacemaker failure characterized by abnormally long intervals (blue intervals) between pacer stimuli. These intervals are longer than the basic interval corresponding to the programmed pacemaker rate and contain no spontaneous beats.

Electrode Misplacement

A common error is reversal of the right arm and left arm electrodes which will produce a negative P, QRS and T wave in lead I.

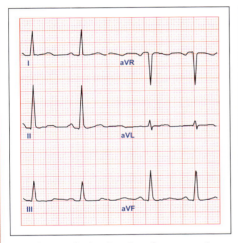

Normal electrode placement

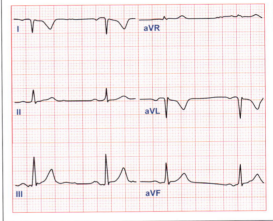

RA and LA electrodes are reversed

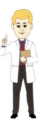

Inverted P, QRS and T waves in lead I is diagnostic of arm electrode reversal.

227

Artifact & Pseudoarrhythmias

Artifact has many causes including, but not limited to, muscle tremors, electromagnetic interference, machine malfunction, loose electrodes or faulty lead wires. Artifact is often misdiagnosed as an arrhythmia and may lead to unnecessary therapeutic intervention.

To help avoid misdiagnosis:

 Look at every lead.

 Look for notches or spikes in the QRS complexes which occur inconsistently.

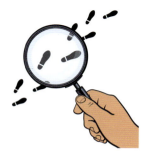

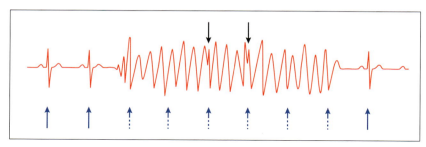

Artifact that mimics a wide complex tachycardia. Note that the artifactual spikes (black arrows) are seen between or within the wide QRS complexes. The dotted blue arrows represent where the QRS complexes are expected. The timing of the spikes corresponds with the expected timing of the QRS complexes.

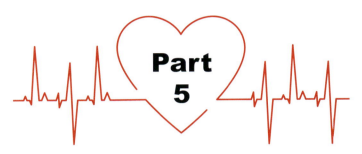

Part 5

How to Read an ECG

1. Calibration

Determines if the electrical activity is measured and printed correctly.

Standard calibration is 10 mm/mV. This means that 1 mV calibration produces a rectangle of 10 mm height and 5 mm width.

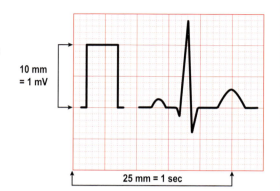

2. Quick Rhythm Analysis

- **Rate**
    - Is the rate slow (< 60/min), normal (60-100/min) or fast (> 100/min)?

- **Regularity**
    - Are the RR intervals regular or irregular?

- **Wave Sequence**
    - Are P waves present?
    - Are there P waves before or after the QRS complexes?
    - Are there more or less P waves than QRS complexes?
    - Are there variations in the PR intervals?

- **QRS Width**
    - Are the QRS complexes narrow or wide?

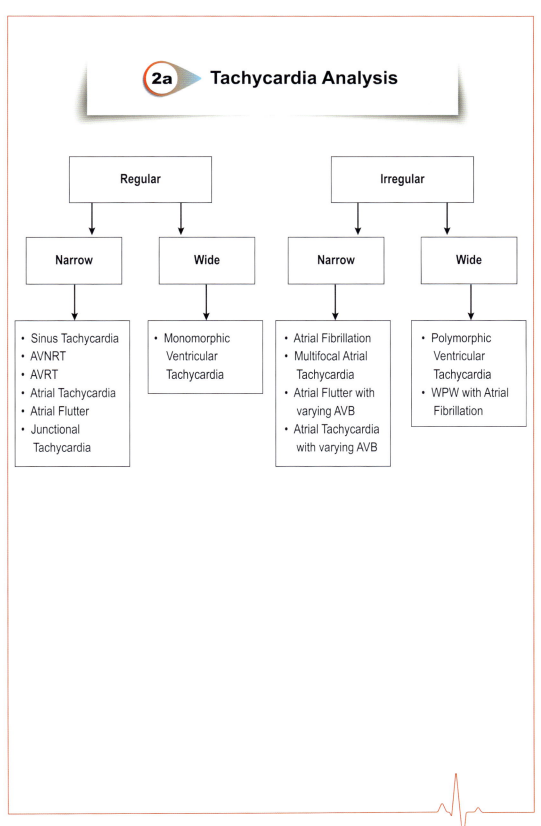

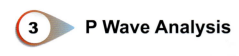

3 — P Wave Analysis

Normal P Wave
lead II ≤ 0.12 sec and < 2.5 mm
and lead V1 is biphasic

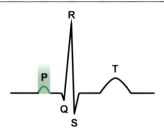

Too wide
> 0.12 sec and notched in lead II and prominent negative forces in lead V1

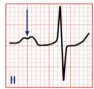 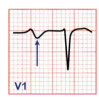

- Left Atrial Abnormality

Too tall
> 2.5 mm in lead II and
> 1.5 mm in lead V1

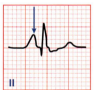 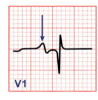

- Right Atrial Abnormality

Inverted
negative deflection

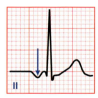 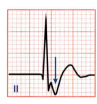

- Retrograde P waves

Changes over time

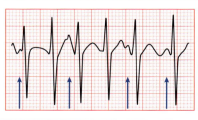

- Wandering ectopic foci?

232

4 QRS Complex Analysis

- QRS Duration
- QRS Voltage
- R Wave Progression
- Q Waves
- QRS Axis

4a QRS Duration

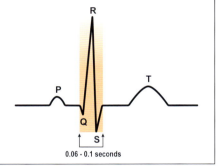

Normal QRS Duration
≤ 0.10 sec

0.06 - 0.1 seconds

Delayed
(> 0.10 sec and < 0.12 sec)

- Left or right intraventricular delay without block.

Wide
(≥ 0.12 sec)

- Intraventricular conduction disturbance (RBBB, LBBB, non-specific block and bifascicular block) in the absence of a rhythm abnormality.

- All ventricular arrhythmias and tachyarrhythmias have wide QRS complexes.

4b QRS Voltage

High	**Low**
S wave in lead V1 + R wave in lead V6 ≥ 35 mm R wave in lead aVL > 11 mm • Left Ventricular Hypertrophy	Amplitude of < 5 mm of all QRS complexes in the frontal leads or < 10 mm in the precordial leads • Pericardial effusion • COPD • Pneumothorax • Marked obesity • Cardiomyopathy

4c R wave Progression

Normal R wave progression

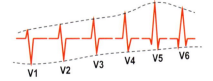

Poor R wave progression

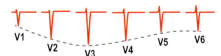

- Superior misplacement of V1 and V2 electrodes
- Anterior wall STEMI
- LVH
- LBBB
- Tension pneumothorax w/ mediastinal shift
- WPW syndrome

Reverse R wave progression

- Reversal of V1 and V2 electrodes
- Right ventricular hypertrophy
- Posterior STEMI

4d ▸ Q Waves

Normal q waves	• small q waves occur as a result of normal septal depolarization seen in leads I, aVL, V5, and V6 • q waves may also be seen in leads III and aVF and are less than 1/3 the amplitude of the R wave

Pathological Q waves	• any Q wave or QS complex in leads V2 and V3 that measures ≥ 0.02 sec indicates prior myocardial infarction • any Q wave or QS complex in two leads of a continuous lead grouping (I and aVL; II, III and aVF; V1 to V6) with a duration of > 0.03 sec and > 0.1 mV deep indicates prior myocardial infarction

4e QRS Axis

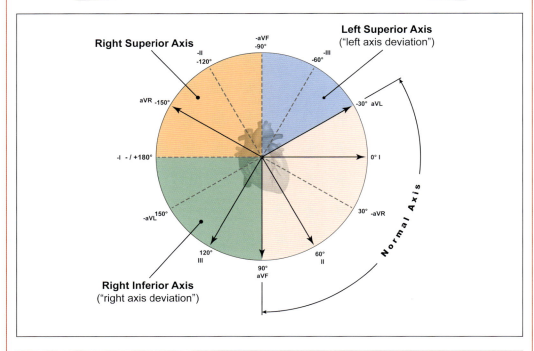
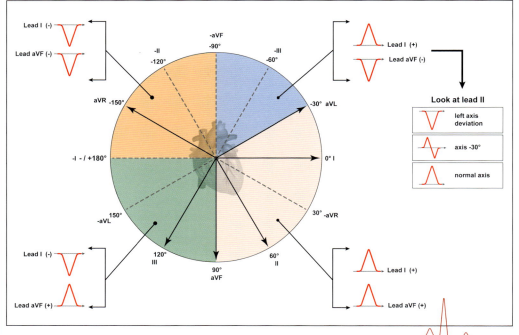

5 ▸ T Wave Analysis

Normal T wave
generally the same direction as the main QRS deflection, upright in leads I, II, V3 to V6 and always negative in lead aVR

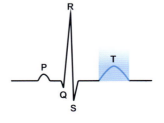

High Amplitude (peaked)

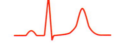

- Hyperkalemia
- Early sign of an acute STEMI

Inverted

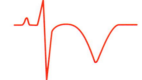

- Acute coronary syndrome
- LVH & RVH
- LBBB & RBBB
- Pulmonary disease
- Neurological disease
- WPW
- Cardiomyopathy
- Paced rhythm
- Normal variant

Camel Hump

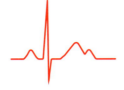

- Hidden P waves embedded in the T wave due to non-conducted atrial premature impulse, sinus tachycardia and various types of AV block
- U wave fused to T wave from hypokalemia

237

6 ST Segment Analysis

Normal ST Segment
usually flat, isoelectric and level with the PR interval

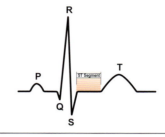

ELEVATION

→ Concave
- Early repolarization
- Pericarditis

→ Convex
- STEMI
- Ventricular aneurysm

→ Coved
- Brugada syndrome

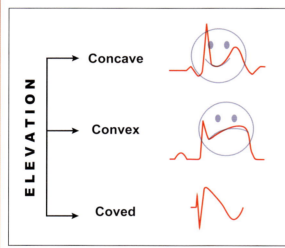

DEPRESSION

downsloping

horizontal

- Coronary ischemia
- NSTEMI
- Reciprocal changes with STEMI
- Drug effect

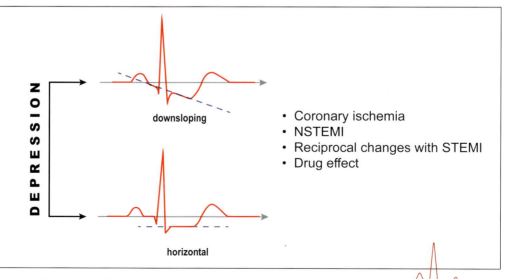

PR Interval Analysis

Normal PR Interval
0.12 to 0.20 sec

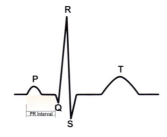

Prolonged (> 0.20 sec)	**Short** (≤ 0.12 sec)
• First degree AV Block	• WPW syndrome

 ## QT Interval Analysis

Normal QTc Interval
≤ 0.44 sec in men and
≤ 0.46 sec in women

QTc - corrected QT interval

$$QTc = \frac{QT}{\sqrt{R-R}}$$

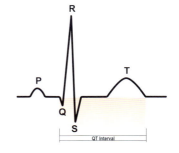

Long QTc	• Congenital or acquired from drug toxicity and electrolyte imbalance

Appendix A

<u>Further Reading</u>

This book can be used as a starting point for electrocardiography. For a more in-depth study of electrocardiography, the following articles and books may be useful.

<u>Specific Topics</u>

Myocardial Infarction
Fourth Universal definition of acute myocardial infarction. https://www.acc.org/latest-in-cardiology/ten-points-to-remember/2018/08/24/00/09/fourth-universal-definition-of-mi-esc-2018

Harrington DH, Stueben F, Lenahan CM. ST-Elevation Myocardial Infarction and Non-ST-Elevation Myocardial Infarction: Medical and Surgical Interventions. Crit Care Nurs Clin North Am. 2019;31:49-64.

Bradyarrhythmias
Wung SF. Bradyarrhythmias: Clinical Presentation, Diagnosis, and Management. Crit Care Nurs Clin North Am. 2016;28:297-308

Atrial Flutter
Cosío FG. Atrial Flutter, Typical and Atypical: A Review. Arrhythm Electrophysiol Rev. 2017;6:55-62.

Supraventricular Tachycardia
Mahtani AU, Nair DG. Supraventricular Tachycardia. Med Clin North Am. 2019;103:863-879.

Al-Zaiti SS, Magdic KS. Paroxysmal Supraventricular Tachycardia: Pathophysiology, Diagnosis, and Management. Crit Care Nurs Clin North Am. 2016;28:309-16.

Wolf-Parkinson-White Syndrome
Kesler K, Lahham S. Tachyarrhythmia in Wolff-Parkinson-White Syndrome. West J Emerg Med. 2016;17:469-70.

Ventricular Arrhythmias
AlMahameed ST, Ziv O. Ventricular Arrhythmias. Med Clin North Am. 2019;103:881-895.

Second-Degree AV Block
Barold SS, Hayes DL. Second-degree atrioventricular block: a reappraisal. Mayo Clin Proc. 2001;76:44-57.

Hyperkalemia
Ed Burns. Life in the Fast Lane 2019. https://litfl.com/hyperkalaemia-ecg-library/

Cardiac Pacemakers
The Basics of Paced Rhythms. https://www.ecgmedicaltraining.com/the-basics-of-paced-rhythms-part-1/

General Electrocardiography

1. Chou's Electrocardiography in Clinical Practice, 6th Edition. Elsevier Philadelphia PA 2008

2. O'Keefe JH, Hammill SC, Freed MS. The Complete Guide to the ECG. 4Th Edition. Burlington MA, Jones and Bartlett 2016.

3. Strauss DG, Schocken DD. Marriott's Practical Electrocardiography. 13th Edition, Philadelphia, PA Wolters Kluver 2020.

4. Goldberger AL, Goldberger ZD, Shvilkin A. Goldberger's Clinical Electrocardiography. A Simplified approach. 9th Edition, New York NY, Elsevier 2017.

5. Stroobandt RX, Barold SS, Sinnaeve AF. ECG from Basics to Essentials. Step by Step. England and New York, Wiley and Sons 2016

Index

A
accelerated idioventricular rhythm 87-88
accelerated junctional rhythm 148, 151-152
accessory pathway 169 -170
action potential 8-9
acute coronary syndrome 111
angina 111
    unstable 111, 120-123
anterograde conduction 14
arrhythmias
    atrial *see* atrial arrhythmias; atrial tachyarrhythmias
    junctional *see* junctional arrhythmias; supraventricular tachyarrhythmias
    ventricular *see* ventricular arrhythmias; ventricular tachyarrhythmias
    Wolf Parkinson White syndrome 174-179
artifact 228
atrial abnormalities 76-78
atrial contraction 4, 5, 13
atrial depolarization 13, 47
atrial fibrillation 158-161, 178-179
atrial flutter 162-164
atrial premature complex 144-146
    aberrantly conducted 146
    conducted 144-145
    non-conducted 145-146
atrial tachycardia
    focal atrial tachycardia 155-156
    multifocal atrial tachycardia 157
atrioventricular (AV) conduction block 199-213
    first degree 200
    second degree 201-209
    third degree 210-213
atrioventricular (AV) dissociation 149, 152, 190, 192, 212-213
atrioventricular (AV) node 10, 12-14
atrioventricular nodal reentrant tachycardia 165-168, 170
atrioventricular reentrant tachycardia 169-170, 177
atrium 3, 4
augmented leads 29, 32-37
AV junction 14
AVNRT
    see atrioventricular nodal reentrant tachycardia
AVRT
    see atrioventricular reentrant tachycardia
axis
    see QRS axis

B
bifascicular block 105-108
bipolar leads 29-31
bradycardia-tachycardia syndrome 171
Brugada syndrome 171
bundle branch block
    bifascicular block 105-108
    left bundle branch block 91-96, 128
    right bundle branch block 86-90, 96, 106-107, 128
bundle branches 10-14
bundle of His 10, 12-14

C
calibration 44, 230
carotid sinus massage 164
chest leads
    see precordial leads
complete heart block
    see third degree AV block
conduction system 10-11

D
delta wave 175-176
depolarization 8
dipole 20, 22-23

E
early repolarization 130-131, 136
ECG
    definition 16
    history 18-19
    machine 17
    paper 44-45
    twelve lead format 41
    twelve lead recording setup 42
Einthoven, William 18-19
Einthoven's triangle 31
Einthoven's law 31
electrical alternans 220
electrodes 17
    misplacement 227
endocardium 6
epicardium 6

F
first degree AV block 200
focal atrial tachycardia 155-156
frontal leads 28-37, 40-42
frontal plane hexaxial diagram 34-37
fusion beat 187-188, 190, 192

H
heart rate 66-70, 74
heart rhythm 66
His bundle
    see bundle of His
hyperkalemia 216
hypertrophy 79-83
hypokalemia 217

I
idioventricular rhythm 187-188

Index

I

intraventricular conduction disturbance 85-108
ischemia
    see myocardial ischemia
isoelectric line 46

J

J point
    defined 63
    elevation 112, 130-131
junctional arrhythmias 148-152
junctional escape rhythm 148, 151-152
junctional premature complex 148, 150
junctional tachycardia 148, 151-152

L

LBBB
    see left bundle branch block
lead 23, 27-42
lead axis 23-26
left anterior fascicle 11
left anterior fascicular block 97-100, 105-107
left atrial abnormality 77
left atrium 4
left axis deviation 60, 99-100, 106-107
left bundle branch block 91-96, 128
left posterior fascicle 11
left posterior fascicular block 101-104
left ventricle 4
left ventricular hypertrophy 80-83
limb leads 29-31, 34-37
long QT syndrome 194
low voltage 219

M

Mobitz type I/II block 202-206
multifocal atrial tachycardia 157
myocardial infarction 109-122, 128
    acute anterior wall 113, 115-116
    acute inferior wall 113, 117
    acute lateral wall 113, 114
    acute posterior wall 118
    acute right ventricular 118-119
    acute septal wall 113, 115
    non ST-elevation (NSTEMI) 110-111, 120-122
    old anterior 126
    old lateral 126
myocardial ischemia 109-111, 120-124
myocardium 6

N

narrow QRS complex tachycardia
    evaluation 172-173, 231
normal sinus rhythm 72-73
NSTEMI 110-111, 120-122

P

P wave 47-49, 74, 232
    broad (wide) 77, 232
    high amplitude (tall) 78, 232
    inverted 77, 149-152, 169, 232
pacemaker 221-226
    malfunction 225-226
pericarditis 132-133, 136
pericardium 6
PP interval 71
PR interval 64, 74, 239
    prolonged 200, 239
    short 175, 239
precordial leads 38-39
    left sided 39
    right sided 118
preexcitation syndromes
    see Wolf Parkinson White syndrome
pseudoarrhythmia 228
pulmonary embolism 218
Purkinje fibers 10, 12-14

Q

Q wave
    normal 50, 127, 235
    pathological 125-126, 235
QRS
    see QRS complex
QRS axis 57-60, 74, 236
    determination of 58-60, 236
    left axis deviation 57, 60, 99, 106-107, 236
    right axis deviation 57, 59, 103-104, 236
    right superior axis 57-58, 236
QRS complex 47, 50-60, 74, 233-236
    deflections 50
    nomenclature 51
    origin 52
    duration 55-56, 74, 233
    voltage 216, 234
QT interval 65, 239
QTc interval 65, 74, 239
    long 194, 239

R

R wave 50
R wave progression 54, 234
RBBB
    see right bundle branch block
reciprocal changes 113-114, 116-117, 119
repolarization 8
resting membrane potential 7
retrograde conduction 14, 148-152
right atrial abnormality 78
right atrium 4
right axis deviation 59, 103-104, 106

244

Index

R
right bundle branch block 86-90, 96, 105-107, 128
right sided precordial leads 118
right ventricle 4
right ventricular hypertrophy 84
RR interval 66-70

S
SA node
    see sinoatrial (SA) node
second degree atrioventricular (AV) block 201-209
    advanced 201, 208
    fixed 2 to 1 201, 207, 209
    type I 201-204, 209
    type II 201, 205-206, 209
septum 3
sick sinus syndrome 171
sinoatrial (SA) node 10, 12-14
sinoatrial exit block 142
sinus arrest 143
sinus arrhythmia 141
sinus bradycardia 72, 140
sinus pause
    see sinus arrest
sinus rhythm 72-73
sinus tachycardia 72, 154
ST segment 63, 74, 238
    depression 63, 113, 120, 238
    elevation 63, 112-119, 129-136, 238
STEMI 110-119, 128
    acute anterior wall 113, 115-116
    acute inferior wall 113, 117
    acute lateral wall 113, 114
    acute posterior wall 118
    acute right ventricular 118-119
    acute septal wall 113, 115
supraventricular tachyarrhythmias 153-173, 177-179

T
T wave 47, 61-62, 74, 237
    biphasic 121
    camel hump 145, 237
    flattening 121, 217
    inversion 121, 124, 217, 237
    peaked 112, 216, 237
third degree AV block 210-213
torsades de pointes 193
transverse leads 38-39

U
U wave 47, 217
unipolar leads 32-33, 38-39
unstable angina 111, 120-122

V
vagal induced block 205-206
vector 21
ventricle 3, 4
ventricular aneurysm 134, 136
ventricular arrhythmias 180-188
ventricular contraction 4, 5, 13
ventricular depolarization 13, 47
ventricular escape rhythm 186
ventricular fibrillation 197-198
ventricular flutter 196
ventricular hypertrophy 79-84
ventricular premature complex 181-185
    bigeminy 184
    couplet 184
    interpolated 183
    multifocal 184
    trigeminy 185
    triplet 185
    unifocal 185
ventricular repolarization 47
ventricular tachyarrhythmias 189-198
ventricular tachycardia 190-193, 195
voltage 7
voltage vector 21, 24-26
VT
    see ventricular tachycardia

W
wandering atrial pacemaker 147
Wenckebach type block
    see type 1 second degree AV block
wide QRS complex tachycardia 195, 231
Wolf Parkinson White syndrome 174-179

Z
zero electrode 32-33, 38